Rising To
The Surface

Helen Poskitt

chipmunkapublishing
the mental health publisher

Published by
Chipmunkapublishing
PO Box 6872
Brentwood
Essex CM13 1ZT
United Kingdom

http://www.chipmunkapublishing.com

ISBN 978-1-84991-804-6

Chipmunkapublishing gratefully acknowledge the support of Arts Council England.

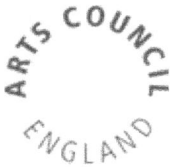

RISING TO THE SURFACE

By Helen Poskitt

To Jonathan, with Love.

With heart-felt thanks to all the friends who helped with encouragement or proof-reading over the years that this novel was taken in and out of a dark drawer.
These include: Ang, Dawn, Ursula, Christine, 'The Helens', Eric and also John O'Brien.

'Obsessions are defined as ideas, thoughts, images and impulses that enter the subject's mind repeatedly. They are recognized as a product of the subject's own mind, are perceived as intrusive and senseless, and efforts are made to resist, ignore or suppress such thoughts. Compulsions are repetitive or stereotyped behaviours that are performed in response to an obsession in order to prevent the occurrence of an unlikely event or to prevent discomfort. Resistance is often evident, but may be minimal in longstanding cases.' [*]

Undine also known as Bubbles

I'm on my way to aversion therapy, yuk! But I've had my hair cut well which always lifts me up, the drastic change to my appearance making me feel like a different person. I look much prettier than I did, even Marius did a double-take when I met him at lunch-time. I descend the narrow steps, being careful not to touch the iron railings in case I leave words on them. Ax notices my hair with a faint approving smile, and lift of dark eyebrows. I look at him, trying to find fault with him and thus inner steadiness. His teeth are slightly stained with cigarette tar, his glossy black hair has grey strands amongst the mane, but the turquoise eyes in the tanned face remain as devastating as ever.

Sitting on the green velvet *chaise longue* I carefully hand over my homework sheet, only pressing it three times in transit, so there's no noticeable delay:

Anxiety Log

	Mon.	Tues.	Wed.	Thurs.	Fri	Sat.	Sun.
Taps	3	4	4	3	4	3	4
Iron	5	3	5	2	2	4	2
Stove	4	4	3	2	4	2	4
Doors	3	1	2	4	3	2	3.

'See, my scores are improving – they're right down,' I say excitedly.

'Yes, they do seem to be, good.'

'Oh and here's the cheque for today, I'll give it to you now so that I don't forget it.' As I turn it over beforehand to check it, Ax's eyes narrow with interest.

'Don't do that, just give it to me Undine.'

'I can't.' I'm smiling, but it's difficult.

'Why not? Why do you want to check it?'

'Because…' It's difficult to speak. He knows this stuff.

'Because I may have written something on it that will be devastating.'

'What would be devastating?'

'Well, I could have written something, lies, about someone I'm really afraid of, and then someone will see it and it'll be apocalyptic.'

'How likely is it that you've written something like that?'

He's staring at me intently, with scientific curiosity and interest. His light eyes sparkle.

I feel hot tears pushing behind my eyes. I'm still trying to smile. 'Very likely,' I say. The tears spill out, my nose starts to run.

'Very likely? Like how many out of ten?'

'Eight.' I sniff, rubbing at my face.

He looks incredulous. 'Eight? Realistically?'

I'm realizing that I've interrogated people for reassurance about my anxieties much more stringently than this: perhaps they felt equally wretched.

'Undine,' he's intent. Rummaging around inside my head with iron tools. 'Realistically, now, take your time.'

'Sorry, what did you ask?' I can't seem to concentrate. This would make a good film setting, the white room, the calm sculptures. The terracotta head on the table has seen it all before. The tears are running over my hands as I rub my face, and push wet fingers up into my hair.

'I need a tissue.'

'In a minute. On a scale of one to ten, how likely is it that you've written something 'apocalyptic' on that cheque? No, don't look at it Undine. In fact, fold it in half without looking at it.'

'I'm not looking, blindfold origami,' I am smiling again slightly. The paper crackles between my fingers.

'Thanks, now out of ten. Take your time.' Silence descends on the room, I feel as though I am under a microscope, spotlit. My mind drifts, while I fiddle with my hair. The cheque lies in my lap. When I touched it, did I indent words on it with my nails?

'Breathe Undine.'

'Oh, yes.'

'So..?'

'Six.'

'So you think that realistically, judging from past experience, you have written something other than the norm on this cheque. Think about this: I may have written something other on this cheque. If I have, it's not the end of the world and I will be able to cope. Try saying that Undine.'

I feel humiliated and ridiculous. 'But it's not true.'

'But you would cope?'

'I'd have to.'

'So you would manage. If you don't cope there's nothing.' He's looking at me sideways.

I know, I'm already onto his wavelength. Death.

Suddenly he says, and I can relate to this: 'That's what I deal with.' It's a relief to feel that Ax can provide a sort of safety.

'In the past, I tried to drink myself to death. I've had at least one breakdown, and after the last lot of flak, I don't know if I could face it again.'

'Well, would you? Or not?'

'I'd have to,' I say automatically. After all, there's never been anyone else to help.

'You can write about it, at least,' he says suddenly. I now feel that I haven't suffered as much as other patients, I'm guiltily privileged.

'So you would cope Undine, you might not do it very well, but you would handle it.'

'Maybe.'

I am having trouble dealing with this totally new persona he's adopted, that of Stalinist interrogator.

'Now think it through three times. If I have written something other on the cheque, it's not the end of the world, I might have trouble dealing with it but I would cope. Take your time.'

I stare up at a beautiful blue Arabic lampshade. In previous sessions Ax has been warm, friendly and calming. I remember reading that a beautiful woman interrogator talked with a Russian prisoner daily for many weeks. She was dignified and demure. Then one day she arrived dressed as a tart and threatened him and swore. He cracked.

I become aware that the silence is still there. I feel very cold, the tears have dried stiff on my face.

'I can't think it,' I have to be honest.

'How would it be if I modelled it for you?'

I hate jargon.

'How about you repeat it after me?' he is asking.

He says quickly: 'I may have written something on the cheque, if I have it is not the end of the world, I might not handle things very well, but I could cope.'

'I still can't remember...'

'I may have written something on the cheque,' he repeats with forced patience.

'I may have written something on the cheque.' It feels like marriage vows. Tears begin flowing again, I clench my fingers painfully into my hair under the bright light.

'if I have it's not the end of the world,'

'if I have it's not the end of the world,' I feel a thud of gut-wrenching disagreement.

'I feel as though I'm being brainwashed.'

'People do not pay to be brainwashed Undine! They are taken against their will and brainwashed.'

It's only later that I realise. You said that when you know that it happened to my poor uncle at that hospital.

'I am not brainwashing you,' Ax says more gently. 'Say it three times.'

I sit there utterly humiliated, unable to remember or to string the sentences together, my mind a grey vacant sea. I am silent, vacantly smiling.

My eyes are hot, more tears wait.

'I don't like you very much at the moment.' I hear myself mutter, I can't look straight at him. I hate him. In my rage I mentally hurl him across the room and smash him face first into the high white wall.

'It's not my job to make you like me, it's my job to try and cure you of Obsessive Compulsive Disorder.'

'You've been all charm, no compassion.'

'Of course I'm compassionate! I couldn't sit here and listen to some of the things I do, if I wasn't caring. I'm sorry you're having a difficult time Undine. I've pushed you through this so that you wouldn't go home and feel that you'd slid backwards, not achieved anything.'

Pause.

'I'm not your friend.'

Ax is just saying that because his supervisor told him to. He's stroked me, he's read me his favourite poem, he's told me all sorts of intimate things about himself. It's a bit odd paying someone to be your friend.

****

Marius

Yeah, I'm Marius, what's it to you? Oh, right. Fair enough. I've been couriering for extra cash lately, I had to quieten down on the other business, know what I mean? When I go to city office blocks to collect a package, if it's not waiting for me in the lobby, I have a laugh with the bird at Reception (if she's not a total dog) then I slip through to the lift. I often know Security, so they look the other way while I ride to the top floor. Makes me feel like a god, looking out over London, seeing all those ants scuttling below. Too many of them. Last week, for a laugh, I dropped a stapler out of a window nineteen floors up – they were refurbishing and had taken out the glass. When I turned back into the office it wasn't empty after all, there was an ugly old bitch lemon-sucking and holding a bundle of papers in the doorway. I heard her calling Security on the phone as the lift doors closed behind me, so I nipped out at the second floor and down the back stairs – didn't want Vince to lose his job – Houdini would've been proud.

Now I can see that the cross of a crane on Park Lane has been decked with early Christmas lights, the crucifix flashing on and off. Traffic, white-lit, fills four lanes scarcely moving around the perimeter of darkening Hyde Park, red slowly-moving tail lights of cars forge a fabulous bauble along Park Lane. (Part of this was in a
poem I wrote a few years back; it got in the prison mag.)

Up here I can just see deserted pavements the other side of Hyde Park. Battersea Power Station's a cardboard cutout, all four white towers equidistant. White and grey-topped buildings below. Along the other wall through office windows, behind the brightly-lit reflection of the empty office with me in it looking the business in my leathers, I can see Westminster Abbey and a slowly unfurling flag, then Big Ben. Further round the room I spot St. Paul's and the Nat West building, the Gherkin, then The Post Office Tower nearby resting on its green glass segmented column. Canary Wharf's concealed behind hideous tower blocks - people on nineteenth floor of same shouldn't throw stones though, or staplers.

Speaking of penthouses, which we weren't, I don't see Aidan any more. Shame that - I enjoyed being his bit of rough. Lately though I can't stop thinking about Undine. Ironic, now I'm willing to do the things she kept on about, commitment stuff – I've even offered to live with her - she's cooled off. I think there's something dodgy going on with that creepy therapist she's seeing. I was lending her money, lending, that's a laugh, to go and see Alexander Swizz. The bastard rang up to change an appointment in his plummy voice, while I was there last week. Just before Undine called it a day, come to think of it. It was as though I wasn't in the room, let alone trying to get her in the mood. And when she gave me marching orders, this time it felt real, like the light that used to be switched on behind her eyes for me has clicked off. She just wasn't interested. Worse, she even started being 'kind' - all that bullshit about: 'It's not you Marius, it's me'. Trouble is I'm having difficulty keeping a lid on my anger – as the trick cyclist inside termed it - it might just spill over onto someone else. Fully malice-aforethought this time. I'm going to pay Swizz a visit. Put the frighteners on and get the money back. He's doing a crap job: she's worse now if anything.

SEVEN MONTHS EARLIER

Alexander had ten minutes before his next patient was due, he'd start on Undine Circumambulate's story. The sessions weren't really working out: she wasn't motivated enough. She hadn't turned up to the last session and persistently avoided doing 'homework'. Undines' fear of rejection would be difficult to deal with, he needed to ask Wendy's advice on the best way of calling it a day. Must remember to do it during their next supervision session and not in bed: Wendy had become unnecessarily hysterical recently about him 'talking shop at inappropriate moments'.

Alexander lit a cigarette and reluctantly pulled the manuscript across the desk towards him. He never read fiction if he could avoid it, so he needed this cigarette. He'd give up tomorrow.

'OCD, A & I
By U C
PROLOGUE

Rosalie halted barefoot in hot puddles of light, to stare through huge windows at Miami's white tower blocks clustered on the horizon. Vivid green palm trees formed a magic carpet from the eighth floor balcony outside, across to the restaurants of Coconut Grove. When she had reassured herself that the sun had indeed risen, that the world had not spun off its axis into chaotic darkness, Rosalie glided across gleaming parquet towards the kitchen. An observer might have noticed that she cast no reflection in the dark wood.

Vampire? I quite enjoy the odd horror story.

As she passed, she angrily turned the thermostat dial: the air conditioning unit visible on the balcony whirred loudly. Every December Greg reproachfully whined about the cost of maintaining a freezing apartment.

Entering the kitchen, Rosalie scowled and grabbed a cloth. She rubbed savagely at a golden stain on the marble table, before realizing it was a ray of sunlight. The ranks of toy trolls on the table watched. Beside the kitchen sink, a necklace lay: a benign serpent with scales of jewels. Rosalie trailed it between sharp dirty nails. The sun smiled on the snake and the coils moved, smearing the clinical kitchen with rich colour. Reminiscent of sunlight moving on a quiet morning through stained glass windows: a veritable church nave. Cursing, Rosalie dropped the necklace, falling back and upsetting a chair. Her long hair hissed around her face like black snakes. Bad hair day, she thought, reaching upward to soothe the shifting coils. Rosalie loathed churches, crucifixes, wooden stakes - all that paraphernalia. Greg, poor sap, still hadn't caught on, and was resentful at being forbidden garlic.

Rosalie looked fearfully at the wall beside the cooker. Behind this lay the swimming pool, let into the central atrium of the apartment block. Not trusting to sight alone, Rosalie went across and sniffed, then touched, the smooth wall with her hands. She was searching for damp. It was her dread to find a crack, presaging an apocalyptic force. The prehistoric alligators circling below in the Everglades, deprived of water by the modern city, yearned for the wall to fall. She knew it.

Greg stumbled heavily along the hall, as usual numb with drugged sleep. 'What was that noise? It's so cold,' he appeared in the doorway, shivering. Rosalie contemptuously ignored him, whipping the necklace round experimentally at arm's length. It hummed above the roar of the refrigerator. A red hole appeared in Greg's grey face, he yawned showing large yellow teeth. His faded hair stood out in tufts; at thirty-five Greg looked fifty. The few friends he was allowed to meet could remember him seven years before, when he had

married Rosalie. They were privately horrified by his decline.
Greg had been a handsome young man; athletic, a party-
giver, a joker – gregarious even, they said to each other
wryly. Benny, Sam and Pete blamed Rosalie for his
transformation. They had been bewildered by his obsession
with her. She was arrogant, she was ugly to look at. But in
seven years, she had slimmed down, glossed up. They
assumed she must have had plastic surgery, the
transformation was so great - particularly the way her nose no
longer met her chin. Her attractions were accentuated by
Greg's decrepit, wintry presence. Maybe that bitch had got
him onto drugs, they conjectured, when drinking together at
Bayside. They missed him. What could they do though? She
had him a virtual prisoner. Greg knew their thoughts because
Rosalie related them to him, mockingly. Now, Greg clumsily
righted the chair lying on the floor, pushing it against the
table.
 'Greg, listen: I still remember the words'
Swinging open the old-fashioned refrigerator door, Greg
looked without hope into the bright empty shelves. The
bloody placenta still bulged in a plastic bag in the separate
freezer compartment.
'Adder's fork and blind-worm's sting,
'Lizard's leg, and owlet's wing,' - Greg are you listening?'
'Sure, Honey.'
'For a charm of powerful trouble' - there!'
'You were the best thing in *Macbeth*,' he grunted obediently.
He clunked the fridge closed with a bare foot and winced.
Fungal sores between his pale toes cracked open and wept.
His yellow belly rumbled.
'I'm going to write a book Greg, but it's going to be a book
with a difference.' Rosalie's golden eyes looked fanatical,
black pupils shrunk to vertical slits. Another craze of hers
Greg thought, running water into a glass.
'It's not another craze of mine,' she breathed menacingly in
his ear. He flinched, spilling the water.
'I'm going to go visit Matilda in London, and I'm going to get
people there to do things I want them to.'
'Like what?'
'Walk out on their loved ones, meet others, become drug
addicts, have children, lose children, die, commit homicide -

who knows? The permutations are endless,' Rosalie said
gloatingly. She inspected her nails.
 'Then what?' he took a sip of water.
'Then write down what happens. A blockbuster – should be
renamed a peoplebuster.'
'Aren't you scared of recriminations, or that people'll sue you?'
Greg was interested. If only someone turned out to be a
match for her.
'Matilda's friends are pretty useless now, they're not going to
be in a fit state to do anything to me after what I have in mind.
Matilda knows some real weirdos-'
Greg intentionally kept his mind blank.
'Who's going to listen to them? What could they prove
anyway? This little woman made me do that? Free will, Greg,
I believe in free will.' She laughed.
Greg looked alarmed.
'They won't let you.' He felt relief. 'You can't go messing up
people's lives, they're not puppets.'
Greg felt sudden fear as Rosalie studied him. He crossed his
legs.

[Alexander smiled.]

'As you've said before, I'm pretty good at getting my own way.
See this?'
She held up the necklace. 'I made it the other day; it's got all
the stones for the different signs of the zodiac. Then I put a
spell on it.'
He laughed unconvincingly; 'Rosalie, you should hear
yourself! Who's weird now?'
Rosalie whipped round, her face hideous with fury. 'You're not
indispensable Greg!'
He ducked, just in time. The necklace sang past his ear.
It snapped with a loud crack and hailstones filled the air. Greg
screamed, his hands clutching his head. Beads smashed and
bounced on white clinical tiles. The Piscean moonstone flew
into the sink, and lay shrouded in water.
Greg brought his hand down shakily in the sudden silence,
and looked at blood smeared redly across his fingers.
Rosalie, eyes staring, stood as though carved from stone.
Her hair sank hissing down around her shoulders.'

It's okay, not my sort of thing. There's a lot left to go.

Alexander shuffled the pages neatly back together and reached for his cigarette in the large marble ashtray. As he stubbed it out he heard the gate at the top of the steps creak, the next patient, Helena, had arrived early. He stood up, hurriedly fanning at the smoky air with her green cardboard file.

****

Bubbles

In real life, whatever that was, it was Wednesday and Bubbles was cleaning Mrs Meidner's large Victorian house at Belsize Park. Mrs Meidner always referred to it as 'Hampstead'. She was a plump, miserly woman with tiny feet and a pince-nez suspended from a gold chain. She walked so lightly that she seemed to float. Now she was hovering behind Bubbles as she obliviously hoovered.
'Undine!' she exclaimed. Bubbles flinched, then plunged at the Hoover 'off' switch with a bare foot.
'Sorry, what did you say?'
'Please, could you not pull on the vacuum cleaner wire like that as Gerald had to repair the plug again this week, and please don't tidy the papers in his study, he was really very angry.'

Gerald was Mrs Meidner's tall, bony, stooping spouse: a distinguished Pathologist of whom, along with her oppressed adult children, she was extremely proud. Bubbles surmised he probably stooped from the habit of bending over to peer at dead bodies. He seemed to dine at Trinity College, Oxford, an inordinate amount. Bubbles had met him only once, when he looked vague and was smoking a pipe, which accounted for all the used brown pipe cleaners littering his study mantelpiece. Whilst scooping these into the waste bin she wondered what distinguished you as a pathologist. More dexterity than your colleagues at carving up corpses? An intuitive, ingenious, but legal, knowledge of the violence used to kill? A sinister interest in unpleasant bodily fluids and pain? It was strange what society valued. Perhaps the college meat catering course had been full when he left school, so Gerald had reluctantly opted for a different career. It made her wonder about surgeons … You could have any scalpel-wielding psycho and with respectable family connections he stayed out of prison, whilst still inspiring fear, even respect. Bubbles became aware that Mrs Meidner was still there.

''Sorry, okay.' Bubbles waited politely until her employer had floated down the broad polished wooden staircase, before switching on the vacuum cleaner again. The thing was, Bubbles thought, staring unseeingly at a silk Indian rug and scrubbing away at the same patch seven times forwards and seven back – she always did things seven times when she was upset, Marius was obviously playing around. Bubbles felt ugly, sad and scared. Well, he must be allowed to do so, who was she to be judgmental? She had an RSJ, let alone a beam, in her own eye. She'd had a couple of one-night stands in the past when she and Marius had sort of split up. She yanked the Hoover round miserably. Whoever it was, was probably so sexy, so self-confident, she would win Marius easily. Better to retire with her own dignity intact. Also, Bubbles tried to reason, she wasn't always sure that she herself hadn't kissed someone else when pressed against them in the rushhour whilst in this relationship with Marius, even though she had made strenuous efforts not to. If she had kissed someone or grabbed them and sort of forgotten, and she hadn't told Marius or always said he was free, she would be racked with guilt that she was deceiving him. It did make life difficult, this slight blurring of reality and unreality, and she would rather believe the worst and have some sort of certainty about things-
'Undine!'
Mrs Meidner was back: 'You've made a hole in the silk rug! I know we want things cleaned, but we don't want our whole home vanishing down the vacuum cleaner.' Bubbles smiled vaguely, distracted by a vision of the house vanishing into the hoover, brick by brick, then the gate, then Mrs Meidner-
'Pop.' said Bubbles softly.
Mrs Meidner bridled. 'Really!' She came to a decision. 'I afraid Undine that we won't be needing you for much longer. I've a live-in companion coming to stay with us next week, I'm sure she'll be able to take care of everything.'

She tripped off briskly to place an advertisement in *The Lady*.

Bubbles looked at Mrs Meidner's wide departing back, industrial strength foundation garments outlined discreetly beneath the polyester maroon dress, then bent to pick up the threadbare duster from a chair. She thought, thank goodness I'm really a Writer. It meant that it didn't matter if she wasn't much good at jobs, or if people disliked her. It was her vocation, uncomplicated by the desire to make a lot of money. (Although, occasionally, Bubbles dreamed of receiving a huge amount, which she could then go and spend on frivolous items.) Actually the writing helped to keep her sane, some of it being autobiographical, now that she'd stopped keeping a diary. Using her daily life as material meant that it never dried up which was handy, and she could usually see the humorous side. One day she would be famous and everything would be fine. Well it wouldn't, because Grania would refuse to read her books or congratulate her. Blinking back tears, Bubbles diligently rubbed wax polish into a bedside table in an effort to forget.

****

Alexander

Alexander had three quarters of an hour or so before Louisa and Lucy were due back. He reluctantly lifted a pile of books off his desk and elbowed out Bubbles's story from beneath them.

CHAPTER ONE
Pisces – water, romance

Horoscope rubbish now.

While water accumulated the other side of the ceiling,
Bubbles dreamt that she was the Lady of Shallott, dying for
love in her boat in the drizzle. She awoke suddenly into
darkness: it was raining indoors. Bubbles could hear an
irregular,ominous, thud of water dripping onto floorboards.
'Murdoch,' she nudged the heap next to her. He grunted.
'Water's coming through the ceiling.'
'It's not so.'
'It is.'
Bubbles slid reluctantly from the warm bed and groped along
the wall for the light switch. As light flooded the room, so did
dirty water. A chunk of plaster fell in slow motion to the floor,
a shallow wave of wet rubble washed around her bare feet.
The cockatiels hissed sleepily from their cage on the floor as
the waterfall from above dwindled to a muddy trickle. Bubbles
rushed out onto the black freezing landing, before realizing
she was naked and risking frostbite of the nipples.
'Don't let her Chloris in here' hissed Murdoch in panic, as she
ricocheted back into the bedroom and warm clothes. Chloris
was an obtuse social worker, who also shared the house.
Her pale eyes would protrude with lascivious glee whenever
she spotted a hapless male. Bubbles now had trouble
dissuading her from calling out the Fire Brigade, while Chloris
donned her contraceptive candlewick dressing-gown. At least
Chloris knew where the stopcock was; it should be her middle
name. Busily, she wrenched up a floorboard near the front
door.
'Hold this Bubbles' she ordered. Kneeling down, she turned
the tap with difficulty.
'There. It must be the tank in the loft,' she conjectured. The
floorboard clattered back into position and Chloris stood,
brushing dirt from her stubby fingers.
'Let's have a look at your ceiling.'
'No. No, I mean, it's stopped now and perhaps Morris can
come and have a look tomorrow, I mean today-' Bubbles
floundered.

'You are being peculiar Bubbles' said Chloris, staring at her accusingly. Suddenly, scenting trapped male, she charged towards the stairs like an oversexed rhinocerous. Her dressing-gown billowed behind. Bubbles managed to overtake her on the landing, and dive panting into her bedroom. Inside, she leaned against the door, weak with laughter; the wooden panels shuddered beneath Chloris's onslaught. Murdoch's eyes protruded above the blankets, like those of a startled frog. The silver plaster Cupids and angels suspended from a huge mobile, swayed in the turbulent air. 'Goodnight Bubbles' Chloris squawked reproachfully, defeated by the lock. Her bedroom door slammed. The birds, Byron and Linnet, bounced up and down on their perch screeching 'Goodnight Harpy, goodnight.'

The cockatiels started up again around eight in the morning. Bubbles had hung the cage in the centre of the high sash window, until someone from the houses behind shot at the birds with an air rifle. She had been donning her jeans when a pellet sang past her nose. A vivid blue Kentish Town sky beckoned outside the un-curtained window, the cheerful light failing to disperse the shadows within the room. The interior of the house was uniformly dark and gloomy, Bubbles reflected. Wondering now why she was so cold, she discovered she was surfing on top of the blue, stained, bumpy mattress *a la* Botticelli, because Murdoch had stolen all the bedclothes. Now he grinned unrepentantly at her, revealing a diamond embedded in a sharp white canine.

Murdoch was pretentious; worse, he pretended to be pro-women. He had enthusiastically helped Matilda and Bubbles to paint Bubbles' bedroom floor with menstrual blood when she moved in. Bubbles was attending a feminist workshop at the time – it had been a good idea, the blood was proving water-resistant. Emboldened by discovering his female side, Murdoch had brought round some of his books, but Bubbles didn't often see him reading them. On the packing crate by the bed teetered feminist ideology by Irigaray, Kristeva, and Moi, topped by *Alice in Wonderland*. Murdoch wanted to see if he could experience genius under the influence of drugs like Charles Dodgson, so an (empty) notebook and biro lay on top. Bubbles' pile of books numbered *The Wind in the*

Willows, along with romantic stuff: *The Prelude, Le Morte D'Arthur, Sir Gawain and the Green Knight.* Concealed by paraphernalia under the bed, were several well-thumbed Mills & Boon paperbacks and *The Story of O*: she had bouts of pretension too. Bubbles had been through a phase of collecting pictures by Piscean artists which was why an unattractive Gaugin etching was taped above the bed, and a large framed Renoir print behind cracked glass was propped precariously on a paint-splattered wooden chair.

Now she wanted to know what Murdoch's ascendant was: 'That's the star rising in the sky at your birth and gives an insight into your character. Mine's Pisces, like my birth sign, apparently I'm dreamy and romantic.'
'I'm Pisces,' he yawned.
'No you're not! You're Scorpio - but I bet your ascendant's something completely different...'
'Sure is.'
Murdoch flicked back the sheet with a flourish, revealing a healthy erection. His grey eyes glittered seductively. He groped for Bubbles' feet and began kneading them expertly: 'That's my stomach' she said with pleasure as his fingers probed the sole. 'This is your thigh' said Murdoch, his voice muffled. Bubbles had discovered that sex helped her anxiety levels, which were off the board. She read a lot too - anything not to engage with too much reality. If she wanted to end a relationship she read whilst having sex.

'I like your pubes blue' Murdoch said afterwards. He ran a long nicotine-stained finger lightly over the golden octopus tattooed on her left thigh. Bubbles clambered out of bed, wrapping herself in a silk kimono from Help the Aged.
'I'm going to the loo. Do you want a cup of tea?' Her breath showed in frosted white clouds.
'No thanks.' Murdoch reached over quickly to pull his woollen jacket further onto the bed. He grinned up at Bubbles wickedly, showing off high cheekbones and freckles. He looked like a pretty satyr.
'Hurry back me darling, and we'll do it again.' His glossy red hair was tousled around muscular shoulders. 'I could wear my wetsuit,' he added tantalisingly. He reached under the bed: 'Why don't you do an Ursula Andress ..?'' He lovingly

inspected the shining knife, running his thumb along the edge of the blade.

Sounds a dangerous relationship.

'Who's that?'
Murdoch looked up at her irritably, 'You've seen old Bond films!'
'Oh, right.' said Bubbles appeasingly. At times like this, the age difference between them jarred. 'Maybe later.'

....

That morning following the flood, Bubbles shut the door carefully, not to protect Murdoch's privacy but because she had a dread of fire. Fires spread if you left doors open. Murdoch had to throw away his week-old cigarette ends because she wouldn't. He'd seen Bubbles peering into the malodorous kitchen bin the day after he'd done so, convinced they would spontaneously ignite. She never cooked so as to avoid rows over washing up. Other neurotic fears centred around needles; dog faeces; intentionally killing people; answering the telephone and causing a fire. Leaving the iron on was a crucial factor in the latter anxiety. She would return minutes later to stare at it, convinced that somehow she had magically plugged it back in. This meant that plugs were obsessively removed from sockets after use, which proved highly irritating for housemates. Bubbles' radio alarm clock also permanently flashed red midnight when connected.

Didn't twig about the needles

Murdoch thought she had problems differentiating between reality and unreality, but it was more than his life was worth to hint that perhaps she ought to talk to someone professional about it. It led to long sessions of cross-examination by Bubbles as to whether he thought she was mad. Actually Murdoch thought she'd missed her vocation as an interrogator: when Bubbles was grilling someone else for reassurance he admired how cunning, relentless and manipulative she could be.

Alone, Bubbles could be found peering under cars and along alleyways, secretly wondering whether she'd seen a corpse and, if so, what she should do about it. She also believed if that if she thought something, this could cause it to happen. This led to her wandering around muttering 'Don't think Bubbles, don't think.' To this end, important expenditure included marihuana, ecstacy, amphetamines, cream cakes, alcohol and creative evening classes-

[Alexander blinked indignantly.] *Is this autobiographical? Undine's always refusing to entertain the idea of medication for her OCD – it might help if she'd try even St. John's Wort while we're working together …*

She was hell to teach due to lack of concentration-

Good self-knowledge!

but was now one of the few women who could ask men back to see their etchings. She often attained a higher state of consciousness than others at the Thursday yoga classes at the Working Men's Institute. Bubbles also borrowed money to spend like water on shoes that didn't fit, but which she hung on her bedroom walls to admire.

She still owes for last week's session.

Previous boyfriends were indulgent, then perplexed, then infuriated by her absent-mindedness. Not to mention - as Sean once said nastily - her metaphorical and physical lack of direction. This was after Bubbles had kept him waiting for an hour at Leicester Square tube station while she tried to find her way there from Covent Garden, a few hundred yards away. Being passionately ecological, Bubbles refused to drive and believed London was accurately depicted by the Tube map. She virtually lived underground in the pedestrian tunnels and trains, as she became lost every time she travelled anywhere on the surface.

Yes, some patients do seem to prefer an enclosed space.

Bubbles viewed the Tube system as magical. She'd been known to ride round and round on the Circle Line for interest and to keep warm, particularly during the first winter she spent in London. That December Bubbles lived in a bleak room in Finsbury Park. It contained a paraffin heater that refused to work until the morning of the day she moved out - when it suddenly obediently radiated a cosy orange glow. There was also a plump Jamaican landlady who hurtled up the stairs to turn off any illicit electric fires if she heard the wheel in the electricity meter on the landing going round fast, and no hot water. Because she'd had a Spartan upbringing in a house with no heating, except in the kitchen, Bubbles stoically accepted this sub-standard accommodation and splashed shivering in cold baths when necessary, as she was keen on cleanliness. Bubbles thought central heating, although sounding bliss, was probably weakening.

The boyfriends were all, bar Murdoch, eventually emasculated by her belief in free love, desire for unconditional love and terror of being loved. Sean had called her a philophobe,

A what?

which soubriquet briefly intrigued Bubbles, before she dismissed it as inaccurate. Murdoch grinned contemptuously when alluding to his ghostly predecessors, all sixty-nine of them. He knew he was a philogynist

Where's the bloody glossary?

and was disappointed to find that there wasn't a slot where he could enter it under 'profession' on his new passport.

Now, on this bright Spring morning, Bubbles glanced fearfully at Chloris's bedroom door; it was closed. Relieved, she wandered down the three steps to the landing window. Her turquoise Moroccan slippers echoed on wide Victorian boards. Peering down through rose-tinted panes, she admired the narrow city gardens shimmering in bright morning light. Raindrops glittered on the laurel bush outside. A floorboard creaked behind her. Elvis, a huge, glossy, black cat squeaked a greeting, before padding down the steps towards her, tail in the air. She bent to lift him but he slid out of her arms like black mercury, purring loudly. Clumps of daffodils and snowdrops shone below outside, amidst ivy and bare boughs. The garden wall, visible behind rampant nettles, was composed of split sacks of cement powder. These had metamorphosed into solid slabs during years of rain. None of the occupants of Einstein Road ever ventured into the miniature wilderness. Cracked black and gold Victorian dolphins swam round the window glass, trapped within peeling white paint. Bubbles swung round dreamily and descended the creaking stairs, Elvis clambered down ahead, dropping ponderously from step to step, his stomach swinging. The heavy wooden banister swayed outwards beneath Bubbles' touch.

Matilda Mugwump, the other house-mate, was lost amid the tribal beat of music blaring from a Marshall amplifier. Bubbles stood in the doorway of the sitting-room watching her practicing an arty stripping routine. Matilda termed herself a 'feminist stripper' which periodically instigated heated debate amongst Housing Co-op members. Now, naked apart from last night's smeared lipstick and waving a long sword, she bent her knees outward, stamping and howling purposefully into the gloom.
'Uh, ah.' Pause, 'Uhh!'

Matilda … Matilda whom he'd treated last year?

Matilda's large breasts juddered as she circled the piano, grimacing. She could have auditioned for Baywatch had she not been so high-browed and low-bosomed.

Yup. Matilda had quite a good voice.

The sword rhythmically stabbed the worn carpet. Panting, she halted and strode across to change the CD, mopping sweat from between her breasts with an antimacassar. Interior window shutters mercifully concealed Matilda from the staider inhabitants of Einstein Road. The attractive new next door neighbour, a film producer, probably wouldn't object though thought Bubbles irritably. It had transpired after he moved in, that he already owned a nude bronze figurine of Matilda. This was one of only three cast after she had posed for the sculptor. One of those London coincidences or what?

A stalker?

Matilda grinned as she saw Bubbles tactfully waiting in the doorway.
'Oh, hi'.
'Is that your new routine?'
Quieter strains of the Radetsky March filled the air.
'Yeah, I was thinking of permanently introducing singing into my act.' Matilda pulled on a striped man's shirt and rolled up the sleeves:
'I sang last night at a Hells Angels' pub in Vauxhall. They didn't seem to know what to make of it.' Bubbles could imagine. Forget biting the heads off chickens, boys, just endure Matilda doing her naked opera spot. Matilda wiped a small hand over her cropped red hair.
'If I move on from the 'Windmill', Dion might come with me. He gets so bored.' Matilda had met Dion on her first evening stripping at the Soho club: it had been lust at first sight. They were both graduates beneath the clothes.

[Alexander rose, bored, and taking up a silver paper knife sliced open an envelope: an invitation to an OCD Discussion. He grabbed his Mont Blanc pen and scrawled a refusal on the form. He peered complacently into a little mirror on the wall and pushed his hair back.] *I'd better glance at the rest of Undine's prose, should be able to get it done by lunchtime. Sordid place she lives in.*

Matilda followed Bubbles into the sunlit kitchen area. Chloris's mother had visited it once, whereupon her gracious smile had switched to sucking-lemon mode. Unfortunately Bubbles didn't get to see her reaction to the stained lavatory, squatting pungently in the back passage. Matilda said that she had stalked out, hi-jacked a cab and roared off to stay in a posh hotel.

Over preparations for breakfast, Bubbles related the drama of the ceiling falling in. 'Did Chloris realise Murdoch was in there?' Matilda asked avidly. She'd stayed at Dion's the night before.

'I had to lean against the door to stop her forcing her way in!' Matilda watched as Bubbles put a soggy box of detergent in the fridge. Bubbles reasoned that if the powder iced up, it would stop leaking everywhere. The groaning fridge needed de-frosting, a fact they both ignored.

'Chloris's written her name on her eggs again.'

'Anally retentive.'

'Can you imagine, if a sperm tried to drill it's way into one of her own, she'd be yanking the egg back trying to autograph it first.'

'Be a mighty brave sperm donor.'

Chloris didn't manage to have sex very often and would jealously lecture Matilda and Bubbles, who did, on their errant ways.

'Sex can put one in a very vulnerable position. You really shouldn't underestimate it, Undine.' she said earnestly one morning. Bubbles had flinched with irritation at the sound of her given name, while Matilda grinned. Bubbles smirked when Chloris, scandalised in orange rubber gloves, plucked Matilda's discarded Dutch cap off the kitchen table. Bubbles and Matilda had decided that if Chloris saw some of their ex-boyfriends, and the things they'd done with them, she'd die of shock. They had also decided that a sure-fire way of identifying women who were connoisseurs of the weight-bearing propensities of chandeliers, was by checking the washing line. The scruffier the outer clothing and the more interesting and smartly maintained the under-garments, the happier the individual. Chloris's underwear not only could have housed several puppies inside each item, but were uniformly the hue of stew. Actually they couldn't imagine anything worse than having a young Social Worker like Chloris assigned to you.

'There you are, in the Valley of the Shadow in a bleak bedsit or a doorway somewhere,' said Matilda 'and snotty middle-class Chloris sails up to you in her Black Watch kilt.'

'Yeah, voice pitched a caring octave higher than usual. You'd just rush out to murder someone wouldn't you?'

'Perhaps that's Chloris's role, to release a nice rush of anger?' suggested Matilda.

I'm surprised Chloris can bear to live with you two bitches. Surely she can afford to live somewhere more up-market?

Now Matilda poured a greasy mess of cold meat stew from a saucepan into a bowl. She propped a cookery book against the flowerpot in the centre of the round table, containing Chloris's *Aloysia Triphylla* (she'd tied a hand-written copper-plate label to one of the leaves). Bubbles watched Matilda practising mind over matter by staring at a glossy photograph of a chocolate gateau, whilst scooping up the stew with her fingers and sucking with relish. Pornography for the taste buds, Matilda being a lousy cook, reflected Bubbles, actually that's pot calling the kettle black. The kettle had expired with a bang after Bubbles had experimentally boiled eggs in it. Bubbles peered into the teapot doubtfully: 'Do you want these herbs any longer for your cystitis, Mat?
'No, it seems to be going, I've stopped using soap.'
Bubbles gingerly tipped the green mushy mess onto the contents of the open bin, and invited herself along on Matilda's weekly excursion to the women's pond at Hampstead Heath.

[Alexander's stomach rumbled. He glanced at his watch, then wiped his fingers fastidiously on a pristine folded handkerchief before removing his glasses – worn only when alone. He rubbed his eyes and stretched.] *Another quarter of an hour.*

Before leaving, Bubbles fed her goldfish in the high dim bathroom. Watery circles overlapped as she dropped salmonella-flavoured breadcrumbs towards the gaping orange mouths. In an odiferous tank on the floor, Oriana the turtle floated with her nose just above the water. She had drowned her male partner. Brown shelves of fungus protruded from the outside of the enamel bath; Dion had reluctantly decided they weren't edible after consulting a reference book in Kentish Town Library. Above the tall frosted window, an old sock was jammed into the sooty fan near the ceiling. Matilda's Dutch cap was spread over the cold tap of the bath, drying: Chloris's peremptory lecture concerning personal hygiene was paying dividends. Bubbles turned on the basin taps, the air in the pipes screamed, rusty water trickled reluctantly into the basin. Twenty minutes later she had managed to achieve a thorough strip wash with the aid of a face flannel, and ran upstairs, rosy and icy, to dress.

Minutes later Bubbles and Matilda emerged from the house into a biting wind. An African man in the house opposite threw up an upstairs sash window.
'Give us a cig, Zoey!' he yelled down to a woman getting out of a whirring black cab.
'Nah, got to fuckin' check wever I got enough, innit?' whined Zoey aggressively. The man grinned ferociously at Matilda and Bubbles. Matilda couldn't decide whether he was middle-class trendy pretending to be street-wise, or whether he genuinely bridged the gap between inside and out. She supposed she, Chloris and Bubbles must be bourgeois, not opening the house shutters to the gaze of passers-by. (Matilda was inclined to categorise where possible.) Bubbles pointed out that they didn't clear dumped rusting objects such as that pram, or litter, from the front garden or clean the sooty house facade - how did she define being bourgeois?

Matilda came from a Mormon family where she and two older siblings had never been allowed to enter the sitting-room, because it had a pristine white carpet and her parents wanted to keep it that way. The parents were missionaries. So far as her Canadian family were concerned, their youngest daughter was an intellectual who had taken up ballet dancing and writing, mercifully abroad. Intellectual or not, Bubbles had read some of Matilda's poetry, which was crammed with hell-fire and allusions to problematic relationships. It was deadly boring.

So is this – at this rate they're never going to reach Hampstead.

They turned away from the Swimming Bath and Public Hall building on the corner, to which Bubbles lugged a black plastic sack of dirty laundry, weekly. Inside was a Victorian laundry room where machines sloshed, children yelled, women chatted - all punctuated by duvet poppers exploding as they were inadvertently fed through the massive hand-operated mangles. Beneath a glass roof, blue tiles reflected the echoes and dancing light of the swimming pool.

As they walked, colonnaded front doorways unravelled alongside them like ribbon. Einstein Road was wide, edged with two and three-storey Victorian buildings, the corner bricks decorated with dappled patterns reminding her of brains. The more dilapidated houses had trees sprouting from the fire walls dividing the roofs. Bubbles and Matilda swung briskly left past the glaziers on the corner, their footsteps echoing from the blackened bricks of the railway arch. Here the terrace periodically cracked up, crumbling houses held up between immaculate neighbours, like drunks between sober friends.
'How's Dion?' Bubbles asked, reminded of his alcoholism. Matilda grimaced: 'He's going to do some street-selling, he wants me to act as a stooge.' This entailed Matilda employing all her acting abilities enthusiastically buying battery-operated fluffy farting dogs outside Oxford Circus Tube, simultaneously keeping an eye out for the police.

Traffic halted them at the junction with Athlone Street and Holles Road. Matilda was smug because it augmented her theories regarding the social divides of Einstein Road. There were builders speeding in grubby white vans, a couple of shiny range-rovers with lethal bull-bars driven by women with bright red lipstick and bleached hair, several cyclists and a courier astride a powerful motor bike. They wandered on past the imposing red and green frontage of The Carlton Tavern, wending their way between black bollards edging the narrow pavement. As Matilda said, if you were wheelchair-bound, or a mother shoving a pushchair, god help you because the council wouldn't. Featureless concrete low blocks of council flats faced expensive cream painted private houses on their side of the road. Here, toys lay in the small privileged front gardens; there, orange notices ordered *No Ball Games, No Skateboarding, Don't walk on the grass* above deserted green patches of lawn outside the flats. Graffiti lit up the end wall of the estate.

As the sun emerged from behind clouds, Matilda loudly declaimed:

The cold ebbs and declines, the clouds lift, in shining showers the rain sheds warmth and falls upon the fair plain, where flowers appear-

Showing off, thought Bubbles, cringing.

'Hey, Mat,' she exclaimed, remembering.

'It's from *Sir Gawain and the Green Knight.* Isn't Spring great?' Matilda began again.

'Mrs Meidner doesn't need me any more,' Bubbles shouted. Embarrassed, she avoided the stare of a passing woman weighed down by bulging carrier bags. The road stretched concretely ahead, as they pushed against a chill malevolent breeze, clutching their swimming towels. Matilda stopped quoting.

'What happened?'

'Oh, she's got a live-in companion coming or something. It means I haven't got any money left until my dole comes through…'

Deftly deflecting the hint, Matilda began enthusiastically bellowing excerpts from Gawain again.

'I pick up the Bible once a week and open it at random' Bubbles said desperately. Matilda was shocked into silence.

'I don't believe any of it', Bubbles said defensively.

'No … So what did it say last time?' They walked on.

'It was *Revelation 22* yesterday. Um, err, 'He showed me the river of the water of life, bright as crystal, flowing from the throne of God.'

'Oh Jesus, it's Mothering Sunday soon,' said Matilda, stunned. 'It must have been wonderful two thousand years ago before humans polluted the oceans and rivers.'

'I'll get her a card.'

'Murdoch says the next wars will be about water-' Bubbles' words were drowned as they passed a school. '- Well at least the clocks going forward will cheer him up. Mat, would you mind lending me some money? I can pay you back from my first wage packet.'

Children shrieked behind high brick walls topped with wire fencing; the barred metal gate was padlocked. *Warning, Hazchem* Matilda read aloud, from a lurid notice on the wall.

'Funny, I thought it was kids.' Matilda often vowed vehemently never to have any. Bubbles empathised with that (as did Murdoch): maternal instincts made fools of women. They should be awarded bravery medals for voluntarily giving birth more than once. Bubbles conjectured that if you had children, your face stayed young and your body aged overnight, and the reverse happened if you didn't. She often experienced revulsion at the thought of all that warm smelly sperm flooding the world. At any moment they could drown in it, the amount of male masturbation going on.

Ugh, too much information!

'Mat?'
'Oh, okay £30! But I need it back by the end of the month.'
'Oh yes, I promise! Sooner in fact, thanks.'

On the rise beside Kiln Place they looked down on a jumble of houses. It felt now as if they had entered countryside: the wide uncluttered sky arching above, their limbs moving freely in unaccustomed space, seeing trees.

The sanctuary of Oak Village briefly folded them round. Narrow roads lined with quaint balconied cottages, lovingly restored and painted. Burglar alarms blinked beneath the eaves, in lieu of birds.
'Do you like Murdoch that way?' asked Matilda suddenly.
'What way?'
Bubbles wasn't in love with Murdoch, but reckoned she could be in three weeks' time. Boredom and recklessness often propelled her towards self-destruction.
'Settling down way' said Matilda impatiently.
'I'm scared of getting too fond of him' Bubbles admitted. 'He always holds out hope, but he never commits himself beyond a certain stage, after which he's slippery as a fish. It's like being with someone who's married - to himself.'
'Just think, you could have had your own romantic isolation tank the pair of you, if the room had filled up a bit more,' Matilda remarked.
'Thanks, I've always wanted to share one with a piranha. Do you know, when he was younger, he was going to be a priest.'
'God!' exclaimed Matilda incredulously.

'That as well, knowing him.'

Scaffolding squared off the 1930s Lido building at the Heath entrance. Balconied Victorian flats stared aloofly above them as they marched along. The council had erected green and gold dog shit bins beside the tarmac path. Bubbles shuddered and gave them a wide berth, visualising faeces leaping out.

[Alexander made a note on a sheet of paper.]

Matilda halted to inspect a rusty bollard beside the fence; London County Council boundary it proclaimed in raised capitals. An empty bandstand in metal and red brick could be seen between silver birches, trunks shimmering like water. She noticed Bubbles lifting her feet to obsessively check the soles of her shoes, but kindly ignored her.

The mock-Tudor mansions in Highgate formed a distant backdrop. Originally homes for distressed gentlewomen, the blocks now pigeon-holed distressed modern women in bedsits and small flats. Bubbles knew this because Helena lived there. She saw with relief the green domed church nearby at the top of a steep hill, they were nearly at the Women's Pond. Other spires shone silver in the stormy light, against purple clouds. An ambulance siren sawed plaintively above the distant hum of traffic, and passenger trains shunted past on the North London line behind them. The BT Babble Tower penetrated the silent sky.

Human din quietened into sparrows trilling beside them in the hawthorn and ivy hedge edging the path. Seagulls and crows were marching stiff-legged across the turf, pecking, as they climbed the sane green slope to Parliament Hill. It reminded Bubbles of her favourite story book as a child, with a drab hard cover. Inside, the worn pages smelt old. Amongst the print there had been glowing pictures of knights jousting, and women in long robes sitting weaving flowers in fields beneath blue skies with white clouds. Nearby on the heath, three barking Labradors jumped around a middle-aged man in a navy Barbour jacket. A few couples criss-crossed the grassy slopes. A blithe modern story book.

Some action would be good.

The top of the hill rose two-dimensional, clean and pure - like
the edge of the world. A wrought iron bench appeared.
'That's like in Death Valley, in America. In the middle of all
this scorching dead landscape, there was a seat up on one of
the rocks.'
'Did you sit on it?' Bubbles asked hopefully, panting.
'No,' said Matilda, striding ahead. They breasted the summit:
London was laid out in silver glancing light before them. The
Nat West Tower blocking in the left of the vista, St Pauls'
Cathedral towards the centre, the turrets of St Pancras
Station.
Bubbles shouted euphorically: 'I love London!' An aeroplane
banked above the heath. Matilda and Bubbles staggered
arm-in-arm amongst tussocks of grass down the steep slope
towards the ponds, the breeze freezing their ears. A
helicopter whirred and clattered above, the sound drowning
their laughter.

A cyclist zipped towards them across the 'No Cycling' sign
stencilled in yellow on the tarmac. Canada geese waddled
bossily along the path, moorhens squeaked on the water,
swans hissed and arched their necks like white snakes
behind the metal railings.
'Come on Bubbles,' ordered Matilda, noting her fatigue with
disapproval. 'We'll never get there.'
'I don't think I'm going to swim,' Bubbles said hesitantly, 'It's
too cold. I don't want to end up an Ophelia.'
Matilda frowned and shifted her towel to the other arm. They
circumvented the black perimeter railings of the women's
pond. The water was discreetly concealed by a screen of
trees; grassy slopes and orange lifebuoys were briefly visible.
At the entrance in a muddy lane, were signs officiously
forbidding the patrons from doing or being a startling number
of things. It ended: 'Women's Toilets 300 metres', above an
arrow helpfully pointing back the way they'd come.
'As if anyone's going to get out to go to the loo,' said Bubbles
scornfully

'But they hope they do. Hope is the human condition.' said Matilda smugly, who'd done inner voyaging on rural weekends.

'I'm not human then,' said Bubbles, suddenly feeling wretched. 'I never managed to get past Chapter One of *She Yearned for Love*. Bubbles mockingly drawled the title.

'I thought you'd almost finished writing the book.'

Bubbles looked embarrassed: 'No, I just thought if I told people I had, it would force me to do it. Moon & Bonk pay so well for romances, well, soft porn. Anyway, money's not everything, evil stuff.'

'Money's not evil, it's just a neutral form of exchange. It's what some people do with it, or to get it, that's bad.'

'Yeah…' Bubbles mentally rolled her eyes, Matilda was off on her hobby horse.

'It's ridiculous if people think that they are better than others because they have more filthy lucre. I've met some terrible snobs over here, they're quite funny really.' Matilda was jumping Beechers Brook.

'Perhaps I could see if speaking to someone would help give me the confidence to write… I keep sabotaging myself, saying what's the point?'

'If you're serious about talking to someone Bubbles, I found a guy in Camden,'

'Yes, I am… But I ought to be doing something to help others, I'm not good at anything though, except writing, and maybe not even that. Perhaps if I wrote funny things that cheered people up on the bus home from work-?'

'Stop beating yourself up. He's called Alexander Swisz, he's pretty good,' persisted Matilda patiently. She knew from experience that at some level Bubbles was listening.

Christ, she's put me in it! [Alexander slumped back in his chair staring at the page.]

'Would me writing funny things help other people, a tiny bit? What do you think, Matilda? To provide an escape from horrible daily reality? And I really enjoy writing, which is pure selfish self-indulgence, so that's bad, isn't it?'

'Alexander was really helpful at helping me to overcome performance anxiety …'

What right do I have to communicate my views? With the fall in literacy I'm an anachronism in my own time … What did you say?'
'He's eye candy.'
'Did you strip for him?' asked Bubbles, intrigued, abruptly abandoning higher thought.
'No, but I wouldn't have minded.'

Interesting!

'Reeally? So where's his practice?'
'Actually, when I last saw him, he was going to move – Knightsbridge? No, hang on, Eaton Place.'

Thanks Undine!

'Mat-'
'What?'
'It doesn't matter. Mat-'
Matilda stopped short on the path to look at Bubbles, who was flapping her hands around anxiously, and waited patiently.
'Do you think this guy would deal with something called OCD?'
'What's that?'
'Just…. Does he?'
'I don't know. He deals with lots of different areas though, definitely Performance Anxiety, and Depression.'
'Perhaps I will see him. It doesn't mean I'm mad though does it?'

Yes, you stupid woman. Thank God, one cigarette left. [As Alex fumbled it out of the box, still staring at the page, it broke in half.]

Bloody hell!

'Do I look insane?' asked Matilda laughing, and privately thinking, Yes, Bubbles is a few sandwiches short of a picnic.
'No… Okay. Will you give me his number?'
'Sure.'
They began walking again, Bubbles's face stiff with tension.

'Stop droning Bubbles!'

Bubbles stopped, hurt. She'd been humming the *Sea Symphony*.

The footpath wound away from the two young women through the trees, to an Arcadian paradise containing the pond. A large green shed stood open next to the wooden jetty.
Bubbles sat cold-nosed on the grass near the water, ignoring Matilda's blandishments. Stubbornly she opened a copy of *King Lear*.
'I'm not swimming: I'm supposed to have done this ages ago for my evening class, leave me alone. No wonder you've got cystitis.'
When Matilda surfaced from the first freezing plunge, Bubbles remembered the way your head ached from the cold shock. Blinking water from her eyes, Matilda swam shudderingly across the pond, then back to the bank like a jerky clockwork toy. Brown water gulped amongst the reeds.
'I'm getting out now' she called to Bubbles with difficulty from her frozen face. Bubbles watched nonplussed as Matilda stood up then fell backwards with an exclamation. She explained later that something alive jerked beneath one heel. Safely on the bank, she clutched at a towel, her sturdy thighs goose-pimpled purple. Bubbles was startled to see that Matilda looked totally extinguished: her face was grey, water streamed from her. Slimy grey mud slid from between her red toes.
'It's disgusting, I didn't realise Gloucester had his eyes pulled out:' Bubbles said, grimacing at the pages of the play. 'I only remembered Lear going mad and the storm.'
A tall woman in a sensible navy swimming costume waved enthusiastically from the jetty. She strode towards them.
'Who's that?'
'That's Diana' said Matilda resignedly, 'I think she's taken a fancy to me. She usually gives me a hand up the bank - whether I want it or not.'
Immune to the cold, Diana beamed at Matilda.
'Hi,' she said heartily. She took a corner of the towel Matilda was hurriedly draping around herself, and tenderly wiped Matilda's cheek with it. Matilda grinned weakly while Bubbles watched, transfixed.

'Who's your friend?' asked Diana jealously.

'Oh this is Bubbles. Bubbles, Diana.'

Eyes watering in the wind, Bubbles squinted up at Diana standing above her, a female Colossus. Between Diana's thighs, like an alternative James Bond poster, could be seen a short bald man pushing a hand mower along the path. He resembled the hen-pecked husbands on jolly seaside postcards. Glancing round, Diana stiffened.

'What a cheek! The Council didn't tell me he was coming.'

'Doesn't look as though he has the strength to me,' muttered Bubbles. Matilda smiled, rubbing her arms dry.

Diana stared at Bubbles suspiciously, then turned to bawl: 'Put away your melons girls, there's a man!' She charged off to confront him. He cowered. Bubbles could only see one woman in the water, and a few muffled in coats and scarves sitting on the bank. Minutes later the unfortunate gardener was pushing the mower timidly between them, staring fixedly ahead.

On the way home, Matilda and Bubbles thankfully ducked into the 'Assembly Rooms' pub. It was crowded with scruffily-dressed men and a few women. Most had shut faces, and were watching football on a large television blaring from a shelf in the Saloon Bar. The smoke swirled to the ornate nicotine-polished ceiling. Leaded mirrors covered the walls, reflections of the clientele shimmered romantically amongst rotund curls and curves of glass. Black marble pillars with Corinthian gilded tops soared either side of the carved wooden backdrop to the bar: it resembled an altar. Imitation gas lamps glowed in bunches of three. The young barmaid resembled an acolyte; Bubbles saw Matilda staring at her pure solemn profile as she poured drinks. There was a hush in the smoke before the roar of conversation began again. The floor reverberated beneath their feet as a tube train passed beneath the pub.

'I'm going to the Ladies' Matilda announced loudly, 'Find us a seat.' Many of the scarlet leather seats were slashed, revealing guts of springs and sponge. Wooden bar stools propped up a motley selection of bodies. The pool tables in the other bar were briefly visible amongst the crowd, fringed lights hung low, illuminating felt Elysian fields.

Bubbles found an empty bench as Matilda reappeared, rubbing her head, face contorted with pain.
'There was no bloody lock, and this woman bashed the door into my head while I was sitting there.'
'Have a drink and take your mind off it,' Bubbles said sympathetically, hoping Matilda would pay. Bubbles adored pubs: she felt completely in her element. The cosiness, the comforting smell of beer, the confessions, the superficial pleasantries, the warmth. Matilda gulped wine while Bubbles admired the golden bubbles rising in her glass of cider.
Bubbles went off to wash her hands in the Ladies'. She looked for herself, peering into vacant eyes in the cloudy mirror. Not wanting to use electricity using the hand dryer – Bubbles worried about nuclear waste products - and being too fastidious to touch the roller towel, she wiped her hands surreptitiously on people's coats as she squeezed her way back through the press of people.

'I was thinking of going grape-picking in France this September,' offered Matilda as Bubbles sat down. A couple of pot-bellied middle-aged men stared lewdly.
'Oh yes!' Bubbles agreed enthusiastically. 'That'd be fun. Would it be OK if I came? If I can get the money together ...'
'Yeah. It's called the *vendange*; they pay you a bit and put you up. It's hard work, but imagine that sunshine'
'And all that wine and all those French men.'
They stared at each other, eyes sparkling.
'Plus it'd be heaven to get away from Chloris,' Matilda said maliciously. 'Let's have another drink.'

An hour later they emerged fizzily into the bright grey light of Kentish Town High Street. They turned back to wave at their two paramours standing unsteadily in the pub doorway.
In a concreted square facing Kentish Town Road, a tramp was soliloquizing like Hamlet to an unappreciative audience of two dour women in padded coats sitting on a wooden bench, and a teenager in a grimy sleeping bag lying on the ground. Lurching happily around the tiny space, impervious to the cold, the tramp punctuated his monologue by waving a green bottle at the white sky.
'Mother Mary of God' he bellowed fervently, breath emerging in white clouds:

'Beckham can't score goals
Rush the bugger, bursh my balls-'
He espied a tatty pigeon hobbling in circles in search of
crumbs.
'Hello pigeon!
The firsct pigeon I've ever seen.'
The youth in the sleeping bag pulled it pettishly over his head.
The tramp squatted down unsteadily to stare tenderly into the
bird's beady eyes. Silence fell.
'Hello little chickie!' suddenly roared the Tramp. The bird
emerged from its preoccupation, cocked its head at him then
ran quickly under the bench.
The women shifted their feet.
'I haven't any bread for you. Fucking fuck off, shite!' he sang.

Tourette's Syndrome?

Standing again, the tramp waved expansively at Matilda and
Bubbles. Feeling love and pity, Bubbles gave him her last
pound coin. Encouraged, he continued:
'God bless you darlin'.
I got mugged in the Holloway Road
I want a wee wee. The pigs,
Police should be in prison!
Free all the prisoners up at Holloway gaol
…It's getting smaller.'
Suddenly the women grabbed their shopping bags with red
hands and hurried off side by side, tight-faced. The tramp
was micturating pure alcohol erratically against a rusty lamp
post.

Concentrate on the sleazy side of life, why don't you Undine?

Plastic bags bowled past at head-height in the wind, large
leaves pirouetted and scraped along the pavement. A torn
poster advertising Fantasia plastered itself to Matilda's shin,
she danced around trying to dislodge it as Bubbles staggered
onwards.
'Bubbles?' Matilda caught up with her and handed back a
letter to Murdoch that Bubbles had mistakenly posted into a
litter bin. Clumsily Bubbles tucked it into her rolled towel.

Eating their favourite cream cakes, they rounded the corner into the blessed peace of Einstein Road. Bubbles wiped chocolate from her chin and gesticulated with an éclair at a red Jaguar sports car parked outside the house. They stared at it, whilst scrabbling in pockets for door keys. The car door swung wide and an exotic woman emerged, gleaming boots first, as though from a carapace. Golden hoops glinted in her ears, Bubbles looked admiringly at her perfect sallow skin, long glossy dark rippling hair and slanting golden eyes. She threw a thick crimson velvet scarf over one shoulder, looking at them complacently.

'Matilda?' she asked.

'Rosalie!' exclaimed Matilda with delight. 'You look great, how long are you over for? I wasn't expecting you.' They exchanged extravagant hugs.

'I sent you a card, but you might not have received it yet. I fancied seeing London.'

'Oh Bubbles, this is Rosalie' said Matilda, hiccupping.

'Pleased to meet you.' Bubbles said, smiling at Rosalie warmly. Rosalie didn't smile back. Giving Bubbles an appraising look, she took Matilda's arm and they entered the sitting-room laughing together, leaving Bubbles to close the front door. She heard their animated voices fading behind her and Matilda filling the kettle with water, as she climbed the stairs slowly, feeling chilled. Chloris must have summoned a plumber: Bubbles could imagine her disappointment if they'd turned out to be female.

Murdoch was asleep, looking angelic. He had knocked his wallet of tobacco and *The Grapes of Wrath* on to the floor. One hand cradled his head.

Bubbles sat on the edge of the sagging bed.

'Hi,' he said yawning. Murdoch stretched slowly, smiling at her.

'Do you want to share a hot bath with me?' She kissed him and cuddled into a foetal position under his arm on top of the covers.

'Sure. Where've you been?'

Bubbles regaled him in whispers as they lay deep in steaming water facing one another. She didn't tell him she didn't like Rosalie because she was scared of influencing his opinion.

What if she stopped Murdoch and Rosalie having a sexual relationship by jealous words? It wouldn't be fair. Bubbles believed miserably that all her words and actions had an enormous significance. She avoided overt responsibility like the plague. Her idea of bliss would be to get through life without affecting anyone in any way.

Why write books in which you identify your psychotherapist then?

Murdoch noticing her tension, kindly kissed Bubbles.
'Your eyes have turned green,' he said with pleasure. He took a predatory pleasure in the way there was always a gap at the top of her thighs, even with her knees pressed tightly together. 'You can't close your legs against me' he gloated now as he stroked her gently. His hair floated like seaweed. He should have been called Njord, god of sailors; he was good at cruising anyway. Or perhaps Noah, except he hadn't provided *The Ark* last night, she had. Bubbles smiled to herself and massaged Murdoch's prick slowly with soap; her hands slid, Murdoch's breathing tightened. He lay back, and closed his eyes. Water slopped onto the floor.
'Is anyone in there?' Chloris rapped officiously on the door. Murdoch's eyes snapped open.
'Just a minute,' Bubbles called, giggling.

Murdoch tucked Bubbles back into bed. He inhaled deeply from a spliff then passed it to her. He massaged her face: 'I'm off now.' To her relief he added: 'I'll ring you tomorrow'. He looked rather anxious.
'Fine' she agreed with assumed nonchalance, coughing out smoke. He smiled at her mischievously from the doorway, then she heard his quick, light, footsteps receding down the stairs
and the front door slam.

That afternoon Bubbles dreamt of Rosalie. In her nightmare she babbled incoherently as she researched Phantasmagorical Alienation under the dome of the old British Library.
'By the prickIng of my thumbs, somethIng wIcked thIs way comes', said Matilda, brandishing a silver sword. None of

Bubbles' friends would speak to her any longer; they all loved Rosalie and she hated Bubbles. Bubbles felt a sickening dread. When she walked into her room, Murdoch was in bed with Rosalie. They smiled at Bubbles triumphantly, lust-tossed.

'He should be at the men's pond' said Rudolph Nureyev disapprovingly, pirouetting beside her at night on Hammersmith Bridge. Street lights rippled on black water below. There was a loud splash and Bubbles awoke.'

Was that the front door of the flat? Alleluia! Don't really fancy lunch now though.
[Children's excited voices and footsteps could be heard from the floor above, along with Lucy's voice calling to them to wash their hands.]

****

Bubbles

The first time I went to have therapy with Ax, seven months ago now, I hurried along the wide pavement between the high houses. A salubrious area, with a composed permanence, resting tranquilly in clear air. A man stood at the end of the road in shadow, when I drew closer he warmly greeted me. He was slight, impish, almost ethereal in the half-light. 'Oh God,' I thought. 'I hope it's not him,' but the gods weren't listening – as usual. I followed Alexander Swisz with trepidation down steep narrow steps into a basement flat.

A beautiful girlfriend, Helena, had a similar response to her new teaching colleague, but with all due respect it's different. Not the attraction of course, or the fact that she has Troy syndrome – too much beauty – but that her object of desire may be allowed inside her clothes but only superficially inside her thoughts. Mine's the reverse – I could almost feel my frontal cortex cringing.

Alexander lounged back in the leather chair, one long denim-clad leg carelessly thrown across the other, suede shoe dangling from bare brown foot. The warm subdued light from a lamp on his desk showed his blue-black hair dishevelled and gleaming, his pale almond-shaped eyes stared at me, cat-like.

'Hello Undine, so how are you?' Received pronunciation, deep and caressing. It's the first time I've liked hearing my name, so don't think I'll tell him that friends call me Bubbles. I realised that I was on the edge of the overstuffed armchair, opposite him in the cosy underground room. I cautiously shifted backwards into my seat, avoiding touching the chair with my hands. My carefully-fastened handbag was positioned on the floor where I could see it.

'Fine, um.'

I didn't think anything had fallen out of my bag. I glanced at it quickly.

'I've got your form here.'

He glanced through the pages he held: 'Thanks for sending it to me.'

My heart juddered in my chest; the form had been quite complicated. It was the checking of it afterwards though and sealing of the envelope that had been really stressful. I ended up steaming it open again twice. My brother came up a lot in my replies, but I'd been careful not to specify what I'd done to him and now had trouble dealing with. Which is an EU (English Understatement) if ever there was.

The form reminded me of a gynaecological examination, the questions were potentially so invasive. Brain in stirrups, here we go. Every question I left unanswered, I was sure was alerting Alexander to prod at a painful area. I was just waiting for him to spout that rubbish they sometimes talk in surgeries: 'Now just relax, [while I scoop out a bit of your uterus with a blade]'.

Silly girl, hysterical OTT language! Who'd be a doctor?

The questions – tick relevant box – were grouped in categories: Behaviour, Feelings, Physical Sensations, Images, Thoughts, Interpersonal Relationships, Biological Factors'. Basically, my life. Including fears, sex life, level of dread, physiological state, body image, inability to hold down a job, insomnia, menstruation, level of aggression, whether I worked too hard, smoked … Blah, blah, blah!

One interesting request was, 'Give a description of your mother substitute's personality and her attitude towards you, past and present.'

I initially scrawled 23 pages, fortunately in draft form. I'm always having to send off for a second application form for jobs, having messed up the first. I used bile as ink and inspiration about Grania, then contented myself with a couple of succinct adjectives on the form proper. It was cheering to realise that some of the questions on the sheets were no longer relevant, e.g: stuff to do with aggression, poor body image and bulimia/anorexia. The eating disorders had lasted for eleven years, from when I turned fifteen. So I found myself writing, 'used to apply', quite often; that was quite encouraging.

Alexander asked: 'How does it feel to be telling your problems to a complete stranger.'

'I don't know [yet]. It's all right,' I smiled politely. The air in the room was fragrant with lavender oil.

'I like the smell of lavender,' I said. I wasn't sure what Alexander wanted from me.

'Oh, yes, I smoke.' He looked up from my questionnaire and smiled at me. For once Matilda and I agreed about a man's magnetism. 'But then sometimes I go overboard trying to hide it.'

'You can smoke if you like, I don't mind.' Get a grip Bubbles! And stop staring at him.

'Oh no, I wouldn't do that, it's not like the old days when psychiatrists used to smoke pipes over their poor patients.' Patients.

I looked up at the spines of the books on the wall shelves, brains theorising about brains.

'I can't help noticing that a lot of the answers relate to your brother, Undine, but you don't specify what bothers you. Would you like to talk about it.'

'No. Well not this session if you don't mind.' I looked quickly at my hands clasped in my lap, I didn't think I'd touched anything. Maybe having them in my lap was provocative, I bravely moved my hands further forward a couple of centimetres, towards my knees. Alexander appeared to be absorbed in scanning the pages of my form.

'Are you a Trainee?'

'No!' He looked startled. 'I'm a fully qualified CBT Psychotherapist, with several years' experience.' He looks as though he's in his mid-thirties, which reminded me in a circuitous way that I went out with Mike who was ten years older than me when I was sixteen.
Alexander was waiting politely, I thought I'd better say something.
'Sorry, I don't really understand what CBT means.' I hadn't read about different therapies in case they triggered off my anxiety. This anxiety stalked me like a dangerous animal.

Alexander explained a little about the process of cognitive behavioural therapy, with the help of diagrams drawn enthusiastically with a black felt tip on a whiteboard. He couldn't find the easel for the board so propped it against the leg of his desk, then moved around the oriental rugs on his knees, smiling up at me as I sat above him. He was almost unbearably handsome.
'You have a very pleasant office,'
'Well, I worked in prison for several years, with my office in the equivalent of a cell,' he said defensively, to my surprise. I had him down as laid-back. Obviously he's had a few comments from less privileged clients. I smiled, visualising frilly flowered curtains at the barred windows, pot plants, a rug on the floor and Peter Sellars in *Two Way Stretch*.

Alexander, by now back in his armchair with a pen and pad, asked me to say the first words that came into my head, then misconstrued my replies. I said 'murder' then immediately afterwards, 'step-mother'. I was annoyed because he said that if I murdered Grania, I would be imprisoned in Holloway. Obviously. A few years ago I would have found his words frightening. Most OCD sufferers, I imagined, were gentle and caring individuals, spending their lives struggling against acting on violent compulsions, the very presence of which distressed them inordinately. But I didn't know; I made a vow to try and do some research when I felt more confident.

Alexander had a disturbing print hanging on the wall behind him, by Bosch. I think it's called *The Killing of Christ*. He saw me looking at it and turned. 'Bit depressing isn't it? My

predecessor left it behind and I've never got round to moving it,' he remarked cheerfully.
'I don't like it at all, sorry.'
He looked at me quickly in surprise, then rose to turn the image round to face the wall.
'How's that?'
'Much better. Thank you.' What a sweetie.

'You've had a rough ride with Grania,' he remarked later in the session, apropos of nothing. I didn't think I had divulged much, though I could rectify that. At another point when I said something about living at Einstein Road, he said humorously 'How about giving up self-denial for Lent?'
I decided to tell Alexander about leaving Mrs Meidner's, to colour in a silence. I supposed it must be affecting me some way or another. I'd worked there for six months after all, a long time for me.
'It's good that you can talk about it so objectively,' he said when I had finished.

At the end of that first session I remember I began to check the cheque, so to speak, prior to handing it to him. It was one of my many fears, that I would leave words indented with my fingernails, lies about my brother of whom I was terrified. Police would then arrest him or me and metaphysical, if not physical, hell would become my permanent address.
Alexander asked me to hand him the cheque quickly, which was difficult at the time. As I was walking towards the door, he noticed me looking back to see if I'd left anything behind. He challenged me on that too, and I managed not to look round again, although anxiety jagged up mountainously in my mind.
'This process shouldn't take too long,' he said. 'I'll be interested to see how you feel while you're not working'.
 With all that stress, I clean forgot to tell him that I'd post-dated the cheque. Marius lent me the money to cover it.
He's doing way too much dealing at the moment so now I'm probably laundering drug money. Surprisingly, Marius is all in favour of me having therapy, probably hopes he'll have a quieter life.

Alexander was relaxed when I asked him questions about himself. I'm so glad he's not aloof or defensive, I'd just get frightened. I was the one who responded abruptly when Alexander asked if I needed him to accompany me to the Tube station.

'I don't think that *that* would make any difference,' I said. How could he help? It seemed patronising and reminded me that I have been alone for ever. No normal kindness or support from family, so that when strangers are considerate it's difficult to deal with. Dad was sometimes emotionally there for me, but too much under the Grania cosh to achieve much. Aunt Iris was the one who helped the most, but I didn't see her often enough when I was a child. As an adult, my relationship with her became very difficult as she persistently tried to force me to pretend happy families about Grania, against all evidence to the contrary. Sometimes it proved almost more than I could bear.

Anyway, on this beautiful early Summer evening I went home to Einstein Road and screeched to Matilda how drop-dead gorgeous Alexander was. Matilda said: 'Isn't he? Did it help?' I said I thought it might. Chloris, as a social worker, would know something about therapy I suppose, but I didn't confide in her.

On the occasion that Grania visited me at Einstein Road, Chloris said afterwards: 'Poor Bubbles, she can't talk to her step-mother.' Grania had kept up a barrage of words, an insurmountable wall against any real communication. Usual thing. I overheard her asking Chloris to look after me though, when they thought I was in the lavatory. That's a laugh, Chloris is so thick and self-obsessed. Our lives never overlap, despite sharing a house. She takes the 'phone into her room for hours at the moment – she's had two mobiles nicked in the past two months - and talks to friends about her social work problems. These usually live in Wales so Matilda keeps an eye on the bill, I get too angry to go near it.

I hate the 'phone anyway and rarely answer it, even when it's for me. That's partly why I haven't got a mobile, that and lack of money. I get really anxious and tempted to say awful things when I answer the 'phone, so end up biting my tongue until it's painful. I often seem to say things accidentally that elicit an offended response from the voice at the other end. I can't deal with that, afterwards I have panic attacks and feel sick with worry. There's a public 'phone at the end of Athlone Road I could use in an emergency. I don't like the thought of Matilda and Chloris eavesdropping.

Grania was just about pleasant towards me by the end of the 'phone call I made this morning. I have to ring her. I'm really scared to, because I need her approval so much and she's usually hurtful or doesn't want to speak to me. She only lets me visit home every few months, for a week-end at most and I have to pay rent. I'm scared not to phone her – which would be easier in a way - in case she tries to top herself again and it's my fault. Iris keeps on at me to make weekly calls.'

Iris sounds a bit interfering.

****

Alexander

Alexander entered his office and shut the door. He sat down at his desk, opened a drawer and reached for the cigarette packet. He stopped himself, shut the drawer abruptly and instead unwrapped a mint from a bowl of sweets beside his laptop. He tensely pulled the tatty bundle of paper from beneath Undine's file, halting to check one of his manicured nails. He observed with distaste what appeared to be rodents' toothmarks in the margins of the pages, and a brown tea-stain on the title page of Chapter Two.

CHAPTER TWO
Aries - fire, war

Good job Undine doesn't know I'm Taurus, or she'd probably write something ridiculous. I'm not going to agree to read anything more after this chapter - I'm not a Literary Agent!

'Good fire Mattie!'
'Thanks'
Rosalie and Matilda smiled at each in the rosy glow emanating from a conflagration composed of copies of the *Sun* and a dismantled wooden chair. They were in the sitting-room at Einstein Road. Matilda felt a surge of affection for Rosalie: she was a good laugh. They had met in Miami the year before, when Matilda had been out there working in a dance troupe. They had got to know each other at South Beach and Rosalie had been great, really friendly and generous, Greg too. Matilda had water-skied, swum, gone to barbeques and parties with them, almost daily, for the duration of the booking.

Rosalie sat back on the sofa, elegant legs crossed, looking round complacently. When Matilda remembered Rosalie's luxurious penthouse, and followed her gaze, she became aware of the squalor of the kitchen. The table, partially visible between the high double doors was cluttered with dirty breakfast crockery.
'It's a great house you've got here, so central.' said Rosalie, tactfully.
'No, no tea thanks Mattie, have you any coffee?'
'Only castrated,'
'I'll give it a miss.'
Matilda tried on Rosalie's black leather jacket: it hugged her body, silky and tastefully studded. Aware of Rosalie's admiring stare, Matilda wandered across to the watery mirror in the alcove. The jacket suited her although she was startled by her fierce appearance: she hadn't noticed how thick and dark her eyebrows looked with her short hair. She absently pressed down a corner of her poster of a Rodin lithograph, which was coming unstuck from the chimney breast. The wall felt damp, she noticed. In the picture the woman's naked body was visible, but not her face. Bit like me, I make my

face blank when I'm stripping, thought Matilda. Rosalie was pulling king-size cigarettes from her shirt pocket. Shaking two deftly to the top of the pack, she proffered one to Matilda. 'You don't? Oh sorry, do you mind if I do? That jacket suits you better than it does me.' She inserted a cigarette gently between scarlet lips.

'Who else lives here then?'

Matilda quickly described Chloris: 'social worker, frustrated young hag, quite kind if you can get through the layers of Damart and half-baked socialism'. She mentioned Murdoch and Dion in case Rosalie bumped into them before she could introduce her.

'Dion's a strange name?'

'Short for Dionysus, his mother must have had a presentiment.'

Rosalie looked puzzled.

'That he'd drink?'

'Oh right, perhaps she made it happen.'

'- And you've met Bubbles-'

'I met her at the door. She looks a little … Unfocused,' Rosalie said disparagingly. She frowned momentarily before flicking a high flame from her sapphire-encrusted lighter. Matilda suddenly thought, Bubbles is such an airhead, she drives me mad. Plus she's always scrounging milk or bread, or borrowing money. Maybe I shouldn't fill in time Stripping, but at least I manage to save.

'It's wonderful to have someone here who's part of the real world,' she said ardently, smiling at Rosalie. 'Bubbles and Murdoch are both bloody irresponsible.' She felt a twinge of guilt when Rosalie laughed infectiously, showing sharp white teeth.

'I know the type, you should see some of Greg's friends. I had to ban him from seeing them - they're gross.'

Rosalie had brought a Prada travelling bag with her; it looked incongruous lying open in the middle of the shabby sitting-room carpet. She passed Matilda a package: it proved to be a pair of expensive trainers.

'No, no money Mattie, they're a gift. I know you like sports.' When Matilda gratefully kissed Rosalie, her cheek felt as cold and smooth as marble.

The fire crackled and hissed within the black and veined marble fireplace. Matilda moved library books from the dusty mantelpiece. Rosalie took 'Room at the Top' from her and read the back cover with interest. The flames flickered palely in the sunlight coming through the dingy net curtains at the large Victorian windows. Raindrops glittered like diamonds on the laurel bush outside.
'Which airline did you use?'
'Apollo, they were cool. I watched Armageddon II lying in bed?'
'I thought you only got your own bed in First Class with them.'
'That's right Babes.'
'Wow. Rich bitch.'
'Can I use the bathroom?'
'Do you want a bath? Oh sorry, end of the passage.'

As Rosalie entered the hall, she collided with Murdoch. He'd returned for his tobacco. He stood still, smiling, enjoying the feeling of her coiling around him and her musky perfume. They stared at one another appreciatively.
'And who might you be?' asked Murdoch. Rosalie steadied herself against him, clutching mock-helplessly with sharp red nails at his woollen jacket. 'I'm Rosalie... And you?'
'Murdoch. Pleased to meet you Rosalie.'
Had they looked up, they would have seen Bubbles, newly-woken, staring down at them from the landing like an avenging angel. She watched, transfixed by jealousy, as Murdoch's eyes slid over Rosalie. Beneath the opening of his jacket, his jeans hung low on sleek hips; Rosalie appeared surprisingly tiny next to him. It was as though they were making a silent pact. Rosalie slowly disengaged herself and picked up an envelope from the bottom step. Bubbles stiffened, it was the letter she had been going to post to Murdoch, it must have fallen out of her rolled towel. Rosalie looked at it curiously, 'It seems to be addressed to you.'
'Me?' Murdoch took it and scrutinised the front.

Bubbles shivered as though someone had walked over her grave. She wanted to run downstairs and snatch the letter back, but lacked the courage. Murdoch shoved it quickly into his pocket as Rosalie smiled up at him again, then she disappeared beneath Bubbles, walking towards the back of the house. Bubbles watched as Murdoch cautiously pushed open the kitchen door; she squatted down to watch him between the banisters as he noticed, then examined, the postcard Rosalie had sent announcing her visit. Bubbles was about to stand up and return to her room when, to her shock, Murdoch looked round furtively before pocketing a ten-pound note Chloris had left on the side. Bubbles shrank back as he came out into the hall, then quietly let himself out of the front door.

'That bathroom is gross, Mat!'
'Well, the house is only twenty quid a week each, incredible for central London.'
'How come?'
'It's a Housing Co-Op, we all used to share a squat? Then we got grants to do this place up.'
'When are you going to do it?'
'It's done.'
'Really?'

I'm with Rosalie: it's not much fun living in Undine's fantasy/faction.

Rosalie shuddered and sank further into the plush armchair. She stretched her slim legs voluptuously towards the roaring fire
'I like that guy Murdoch.'
'When did you meet him?'
'Just now in the hall.'
'Was Bubbles there?'
'No.
A topless model flared into orange flame, then blackened in the grate.
 'Anyway, what's been happening? Are you still with Greg? How's the Florida Oranges business? You didn't say much in your card.'
'What's wrong with your email? I sent you a couple of messages just before I came over, but they bounced back.'
'Oh, sorry, I belong to an arts web site and they flood my inbox, I must sort it out. Are you and Greg okay?'
'Let's just say things have been a bit difficult lately.' Rosalie looked strained.

'Oh,' Matilda reached to touch Rosalie's arm sympathetically. 'I'll tell you about it later?'

'Any time, Rosie. I guess the oranges trade is booming, though they're a bit healthy for me.'

'Oh me too, but he does trade other, more unhealthy, stuff.'

'Reeally? Pity you couldn't have brought some.'

'Mm-mh. Come out and see me and we'll have a lost week. Do you remember Coconut Grove?'

They laughed, and launched into reminiscence. An hour later Rosalie stretched, yawning. Her rings cut the air with white light.

'Are those real diamonds?'

'Yes, Greg gave me this one soon after we met.' She held her hand out towards Matilda, palm down, and pulled at a three-carat diamond on her middle finger with her thumb.

'God, why do I always attract losers?' Matilda held Rosalie's hand, inspecting the ring enviously. 'Dion could just about manage something from Argos on a good day.'

'That's a neat poster, where can I get one?' Rosalie moved away across the room to inspect a brightly-coloured Miró print hanging above the oak sideboard.

'Oh,' she said, annoyed, 'It comes from France, that wasn't on my itinerary.'

'How do you know?'

'Because I planned my visit. Oh right. It says on the edge: 'For Tristan Tzara (April 4 1948) Paris.'

'You can tell I'm into my surroundings, not. We might be able to get you one from a gallery.'

Rosalie was getting bored.

'Tell you what Mat, why don't you show me London? The sun's out now.'

'Oh, OK.' said Matilda reluctantly. She'd thought, having lit the fire that they could stay in.

'Do you want to drive?' offered Rosalie cunningly.

'I'd love to – are you sure?'

'Yeah. I'd like to take in some culture - how about we visit that War Museum?'

'Well, I went there last week-end, would you mind if we did the Tate today? We could look for your poster.'

As they emerged from the house, they saw a rainbow above the buildings opposite. A robin stood cheekily on the front of

the hired car like a logo. Rosalie looked back appreciatively at the peeling studded front door as Matilda closed it.
'It's real mediaeval. You'd need a battering ram to get in if you forgot your keys.'
'Bubbles did one night. She got all these hunky firemen to break a window for her. Chloris was in heaven.'
'I'll bet. Those poor guys.'
The interior of the car smelt of new leather and luxury. Matilda took the keys and bent to pick up a CD from the floor.
'Oh chuck that into the front compartment or somewhere.'
Matilda put *Dr Faustus* into the glove compartment.
'What's that smell of smoke?' she asked, clicking closed her seat belt with anticipation. 'I haven't started the engine.'
'Oh, don't worry, probably the air-freshener.'

Sunlight glinted from the glass and metal of other vehicles and the appreciative stares of their drivers as Matilda and Rosalie purred past Mornington Crescent tube station.
'The Underground, what an awful way to travel!' said Rosalie, 'Thank god I hired the car.'
'I was standing on the Tube once,' said Matilda reminiscently. 'It was a boiling hot summer's day, in the rush hour, and I felt this heavy period suddenly come on. I was wearing this long white summer dress and by Camden Town station I looked as though I'd been in a road accident. I kept thinking, 'It's natural, it's natural'. It was traumatic though.'
'Of course it's natural,' Rosalie said indignantly.
'Yeah, people boil hen's periods daily. Hey, what a gas going on a Bleed March would be - soon bring the price of tampons down.'

Bloody feminists

Rosalie was peering into a shop. 'I fancy one of those flame-grilled kebab things, park up Mattie.'

They turned right into the hectic traffic of Euston Road, Rosalie neatly eating a donor kebab, held between sharp red fingernails.
'Hell!' Matilda exclaimed angrily as a lorry roared past a centimetre from the wing mirror.

Rosalie flicked a middle finger at the driver: 'Swivel' she called.

'Pink fluffy feminine, that's was my New Year Resolution Rosalie – like Bubbles.'

'Really?'

'No.' They both laughed.

'Why do parents here shove their kids into the road without looking?' Rosalie asked. She negligently dropped her crumpled kebab paper out of the window into the lap of a toddler in a buggy as the traffic surged forwards, while Matilda was concentrating on avoiding the car in front.

'Think Darwin – it stops the spread of social inadequates... His bloody brake lights don't work! Sorry, what are your plans while you're here?'

Alerted by a sudden silence, Matilda glanced sideways.

'S'okay... I think Greg's having an affair.'

'Oh, Rosalie!'

'It's all right,' said Rosalie, bravely. She dabbed delicately at her eyes under her Ray-bans with a miniscule tissue. 'But I needed to get away.'

'Of course you did.' They dribbled along helpless in the queue of traffic past Great Portland Street station, then accelerated past the stucco curve of Park Crescent.

'And I think I might be pregnant.'

The car stalled at a green traffic light. 'Oh bugger. Is that good news?' asked Matilda carefully, re-starting the engine. A taxi driver glared then began to overtake as they lurched forward.

'I'd love to be.'

'Right' said Matilda, stunned. The taxi driver leaned on his horn and said something pithy over his shoulder to his voluptuously pregnant passenger. She smiled sympathetically.

'Hey, that looks like Helena – Helena!' Matilda called out of the window. The young woman in the back of the cab stared, then waved.

'She's pretty,' said Rosalie jealously.

'You think so?'

'Anyway,' said Rosalie dismissing Helena, 'I've worked out that I can take care of the baby on my own, if I have to. I can always sell my rings.' She sniffed delicately.

'Well, you can stay with me as long as you like,' said Matilda in a spasm of love and generosity. She hurriedly pushed away the thought of the Co-Op members' disapproval. Long-term guests weren't welcome, children were forbidden.
'Oh thank you darling,' said Rosalie tucking away her tissue. Unseen by Matilda, who was overtaking a double-decker bus, Rosalie smiled triumphantly.
'Come on Mat, let's burn off that Porsche!'
In the grip of devilment, they roared through a red light, almost killing a short bald man who worked for Camden Parks department, who was crossing Langham Place.
'Women drivers,' Bert muttered angrily, already upset by his humiliating treatment from Diana earlier that morning. He wandered homeward to Edna, who was washing clean net curtains in their pristine Council flat.

Bubbles was composing poetry in the kitchen at Einstein Road. Although she hadn't added coal, the fire still glowed redly in the sitting-room. She scrawled 'Jealousy' in large script in an exercise book, then -

There was the girl in the hall
The man in her mind.

We looked at her
Smiling pleased, self-conscious
Smoothing down
windblown skirt with her hand,
A venomous Marilyn.

Their glances below me
All in silence, and his smooth pleased face
as he left the house.

I and he no more.

'Bugger Murdoch!' she said with an effort, then crumpled into angry tears.
(At that moment, across town, Aidan was tenderly soaping Murdoch's back in the shower.)

She talks about her boyfriend quite a lot. What's his name, Marcus? Matthew?

As Rosalie and Matilda swung round Eros at Piccadilly Circus, a seagull dumped guano on the car windscreen from a great height. Unable to park they swerved erratically along Horse Guards Road, Rosalie leaning out of the window trying to clear the glass with a sponge, laughing. She cursed the seagull, which obediently flew into an office window and dropped three floors like a stone, narrowly missing a manager enjoying a cigarette break outside the entrance. Matilda turned on the windscreen wipers, guano and glass cleaner sprayed right and left, missing Rosalie and splattering a motorbike courier. Pursued by the furious biker from *Hells Messengers* they sped south, towards the Thames and Tate.

Matilda revved up and slowed down between traffic lights along Vauxhall Bridge Road, the biker boxed in impotently one set of lights behind her.
'Clever liars give details, but the cleverest don't' – I don't know who said it, but the guy I saw before Dion was like that.'
Matilda turned her head to look at Rosalie.
'That's Greg to a "T". I mean, it's great living in Coconut Grove, but I could afford just as good an apartment of my own in Key Biscaine. I wish I'd never bothered with the little jerk!' Rosalie said viciously.
'That's right girl, his loss,' said Matilda loyally, looking idly out of the window at Bessborough Street.

Matilda remembered the feeling of Aidan leaning warmly over her as she knelt on all fours. He had reached down round to her front with tentative fingers, feeling the swell of her breasts above and below the thick leather belt, 'Tighten it' Matilda had ordered, arching her back.'

[Alexander shifted in his seat.]

Aidan whimpered in ecstasy'-

[The doorbell shrilled loudly. Alexander swore, fumbled the pages closed and leapt guiltily to his feet. He tried to shove the manuscript into a drawer, but it was too bulky. He hurled it into a corner, before hurrying across the room to open the door.]

****

Bubbles

Bubbles was newly-employed; Matilda had been offered the job by an actor friend but had turned it down, passing it on to her. She didn't *think* Bubbles could screw it up: it was so simple, unless of course she merely decided not to show up. The journey was a pain, but if you travelled south-west on the North London line you usually got a seat, which beat having your head jammed into someone's armpit on the Tube.

A small boy stared up at Bubbles through watery blue eyes, open-mouthed. Bright green snot welled in one nostril. His mother smiled happily. The child's legs wobbled under him and he grabbed Bubbles's trousers, almost falling. The material pulled against the back of her knee stiffly, she remained motionless with difficulty. The mother prised open the toddler's fingers and lifted him back, smiling up at Bubbles apologetically. As he opened his mouth to roar indignantly, Bubbles bent stiffly and proffered him a promotional voucher. His mouth remained open, but silently, showing two white teeth. She straightened stiffly, staring ahead. Nothing much happened for a while. The lunch-time crowds of office workers drifted or hurried past. Bubbles stared unblinkingly at the toys in the windows of the Dinzey store opposite. Although she told herself that they were designed by anxious adults, made by children for children, she coveted them.

Bit like some of the kids who live round here, she thought, babies made by children. An incandescently pale teenager walked past, carefully pushing an infant, clad in a minute biker's jacket, asleep in a buggy. Wonder if she's from the Guinness Estate? The girl halted briefly, shoulders hunched, to look at baby clothes on special offer behind a shop window. When Bubbles had been her age - only a few years back, but it felt like, and was, a different century - and lived in a tiny bedsit in Oxford, men had followed her home through the darkness along Iffley Road, whispering lewdly. Other men

kerb-crawled in idling cars. Her heart would sink as she
hurried along, hearing the engine slow, the window being
lowered. One night, a policeman did a U-turn in his Panda
car and tried to force her into it. Failing, he furiously revved
away, skidding into the road where she lived. Bubbles,
breathless with fear, jabbed her key into the front door lock,
praying he wasn't hiding down beside the dark steps. Now
she could see cheap linen displayed in a shop out of the
corner of her eye. During silent hours of insomnia in the
bedsit, she'd sat cross-legged on the floor hand-stitching
patchwork quilts.

Bubbles was relieved to be distracted by an attractive middle-
aged woman appearing in her line of vision. The woman
turned to look back at someone, saying unhappily: 'I don't
know what to wear, perhaps my blue silk shirt ... You haven't
seen that –'.
'I've seen everything in your wardrobe,' said someone
arrogantly.
The speaker now appeared, with another man. He was
young, dark-haired and plump, voracity glinting through a
veneer of wealth. He glanced at Bubbles indifferently, then
fell back into conversation with his male companion. His
friend was handsome with light-green eyes, but dissipation
blurred his features. He stared at Bubbles knowingly as he
passed. She cringed inwardly, fighting the urge to check he
had moved on and wasn't standing motionless behind her.

Bubbles stiffened her jaw, trying not to yawn, staring blankly
at the traffic streaming past the Mall entrance. A handsome
Arabic man pulled up in a new white Mercedes, a young
woman in clean but faded clothing clambered out quickly,
pulling a bag behind her. The man said something out of the
open window which halted his passenger's departure. She
looked reluctantly into her backpack. His head bent in turn,
as he searched in the glove compartment, found a pen, then
wrote urgently on a white serviette leaning on the windowsill.
He reached out of the car and pushed the paper pleadingly
into the woman's hand. He stared after her as she walked
quickly towards Bubbles, before pulling out slowly into the
river of traffic. As the woman strode past Bubbles she
dropped the scrap of paper onto the tiled floor. Later, when it

had been trodden into a brown rag, a bored African in a fluorescent tabard lethargically swept it into a long-handled dustpan, along with cigarette butts and a sweet wrapper.

Perhaps because of this incident, Bubbles stepped down to try and help a young man who was holding up the torn bib of his denim dungarees and weeping quietly from an averted face.
'Can I help?' Bubbles asked. The teenager's wet eyes widened momentarily. He tried to wipe away streaks of black mascara with a plump finger, his long chestnut hair rippled around his soft face. 'No. Thank you. I must look a fright.'
'No you don't. What's the matter?'
'You're very kind,' he said, but hurried on. Bubbles heard him sobbing uncontrollably in the distance, still clutching the dungaree bib to his chest.

She would have to stop soon, she was becoming tired. Where was Vic with her money? That was the only drawback of this job, he was sometimes late. Bubbles's legs ached, she felt stiff and would soon begin to tremble. She liked Vic though, he was friendly without being lecherous. A family of Italians clustered before her; a boy reached up to tentatively touch her hand, Bubbles swung it gently. They exclaimed and laughed. A girl took a photograph of her. The mother threw some coins into the box at Bubbles' feet, so Bubbles pretended to shoot some footage of the family with an old movie camera and handed out vouchers.

On Monday, a school-boy had walked over and punched her in the side. Bubbles hadn't responded at the time. She'd seen him yesterday though, and in retaliation for the sleepless nights, had tripped him surreptitiously as he ran past to catch up with his friends. He's fallen heavily into the Cookie stall, rocking the wooden structure so that the bright striped awning flapped perilously and biscuits ricocheted off passers-by. Bubbles had silently smiled, causing the golden mask to crack from side to side.

****

Therapy Session

Is that my book, splayed out across the carpet in the corner
of his office?

Following my stare, Alexander looked indifferently at the
scruffy manuscript, then with a rueful smile he swooped to
pick it up, marshalling the pages neatly with his fingers and
placing it reverently on the desk.

'Sorry Undine, it fell down when a patient got a bit ...
overwrought. I'm so sorry, I didn't have time to tidy up before
your appointment.'

'Oh no, it's OK, fine... I don't suppose you've had time to
read it all yet ?'

'No. I wanted to say - thank you for showing me your work,
but I won't have time to read much more. I'll just check, I
mean read, the rest of the second chapter, then I will let you
have it back.'

'Oh.' Alexander's pristine white shirt emphasises his tan.

'So Undine, how's working again? You said you have a new
job at a shop in, where was it? South Molton Street?'

'Oh, I will soon, but at the moment I'm working as a statue.'
Alexander blinked.

'Oh yes,' I elucidated: 'It's not what I want, because I really
want to write, or draw, but the money's quite good. And it's
interesting material for my novel.'

'How have you been getting on with your book?' He asked
this rather oddly.

'I'm not writing the astrological one any more,' Alex seemed
relieved, I wondered why. 'I was getting a bit stuck on the
'Taurus' chapter – anyway I was giving away too much.'

'Aah, I wondered if it was auto-?'

I looked at Alex enquiringly as he stopped abruptly.

'Alexander, do you think I've been writing the book as a
controlling thing?'

'What do you mean?'

'Rosalie, she's really visiting and she wasn't friendly when we
met, I don't think she likes me. I've only seen her a couple of
times, she's out a lot. Do you think I'm writing it because I
feel threatened by her?'

'Do you?'

'I don't know, I felt awful when she didn't like me.'

'What makes you think she doesn't like you?'

'Because she looked hostile and didn't say 'Hello' when we were introduced. I was being friendly.'

'It's good to be aware if you're mind-reading or script-writing in real life Undine, something to guard against. We don't know what Rosalie was thinking when she met you. What else could have been happening for her?'

'I don't know.'

'Had she just travelled a long way?'

'Yes,' I said.

'So..?'

'She might have been tired or jet-lagged? But she didn't look tired! And she was so warm towards Matilda.'

'Matilda's her friend. Perhaps she's shy?'

'Huh, she didn't look it.'

'Sometimes people through no fault of their own remind people of others that they really don't like. I found myself avoiding a man at a party recently.'

'Why?'

'Because he reminded me of a teacher at school, who used to bully me. Once I realised what was going on, I went over to talk to him.'

'And was he nice?'

Alexander laughed: 'A bit boring actually. Anyway, back to you. You don't know what was going on in Rosalie's mind.'

I felt myself relaxing slightly. The 'phone on the desk next to him pealed suddenly, Alex reached hurriedly to silence it, knocking my manuscript back on to the floor.

'Sorry about that Undine, I was sure I'd put the answerphone on. Look, let me give you this bit back, in case anything else happens to it while it's here. I'll finish the second chapter as soon as I can.' Alex's dark hair fell forward, as he hurriedly handed the pages across to me. Our fingers touched briefly and I visualised the Sistine Chapel ceiling. I placed the manuscript carefully on the carpet by my chair, a centimetre from my coat. My hand tingled from his touch,

'You were saying, about giving away things in your writing - to whom in particular Undine?'

You. I studied the white wall mutely.

'What did you think of the book?' I asked, partly to fill the silence.

My silver eyebrow-stud suddenly hurt – I must have been nervously twisting it for a while.

'Well, I have to say that I didn't really like any of the characters except Bubbles, whom I assume was partly based on you yourself?'

I nodded slowly; inside I felt a warm glow.

'Um, I did think that perhaps Bubbles and Rosalie are, fictionally, the two sides of you.'

'Wow, I should have picked that up.'

'Well it's not always easy to see the wood for the trees when it's one's own writing. By the way I like the fact that you used a fountain pen, they're lovely to write with aren't they?'

....

'I was depressed this week, more so than usual, I think,' I tried to keep my tone light. 'I couldn't stop thinking about the awful or embarrassing things I've done in the past - and how few friends I've got and how many people hate me, including my step-mother and my brother. I've got awful insomnia.'

Alexander made a quick note on his pad.

'When patients have depression, all compassion towards self just vanishes.'

'We're talking about Obsessive Compulsive Disorder,' I reminded him hesitantly.

'Yes, but the two are often linked. It makes it worse if you try too hard to sleep, doesn't it? Well, don't forget if you're lying down, you're still resting physically. Or you can ...'

I feel so relaxed sometimes when listening to his voice, that I could just slide into sleep during one of our sessions. Perhaps I should just ask Alex to come round and talk me to sleep. I think we might hit a reality check if he ever laid eyes on the Gothic Manse though, when he's used to luxurious surroundings like these. Perhaps a CD -

'Undine, I feel you're drifting, do you want to tell me what you're thinking about?'

'No, nothing,' I said hurriedly, sitting upright.

....

'Um, I saw this guy outside the cinema, that I fancied ... '

Alex waited.

'I don't know if I touched him, when I walked past him as I was leaving.'

'How do you mean, touched him?'

'Well, sexually.' I was hot-faced and tense.

'Does it matter if you did?'

'Yes, no- Well, I'm supposed to be seeing Marius. I know,' I said with a mixture of misery and relief, 'I can chuck him and then it won't matter if I've been unfaithful. Or I'll say that I can sleep with who I like and so can he, and then say I already have - just to be on the safe side.'

'Have you?'

'I don't know.' I felt sick. There was silence, I stared at Alexander.

'How would you feel about having an open relationship like that with Marius?'

'I could manage, it would stop my worries. Anyway, other people have them all the time, so I should be able to cope'.

'Whether they do or don't isn't relevant.'

'Isn't it?'

'No. We're talking about you.'

'If Marius was unfaithful, I'd feel terrible.' That was the first time I'd ever said it aloud. 'I feel as though I'm being unfaithful if I even look at someone else,' I said.

'How about seeing it as just nature's way of increasing the gene pool?'

'You're married aren't you? Is that what you do?'

'We're not talking about me. But yes,' Alexander conceded after a pause. So he is married.

'By the way,' he said, his light eyes beautiful with laughter, 'did you know that women are most fertile and randy a few months after giving birth, and attract different men? It's Nature's way of ensuring that all the litter don't exist from the same genes, in case they're weak.'

'Wow, you wouldn't want to publicise that … So, it's only Nature's way of increasing the gene pool?'

'Yes, it's normal to look at others in that way, it's even okay to fantasise.'

I felt my clenched stomach relax, and warmth and safety enfold me for a second.

'I do have other worries about this, can I talk about it another time?'

'Yes. Now, how did you get on with the homework?'

'We can really talk about my worries another time?
'Yes,' Alexander repeated with forced patience.
'Sorry, I haven't done any homework. I didn't have time.'
There was silence. I felt myself blushing again as Alex looked at me coldly.
'I feel there's some resistance here,' he said slowly. 'I want you to think about whether that's
advantageous.'
His mobile rang, saved by the bell.
'Sorry,' he muttered, leaning back in his chair and fishing in his jeans pocket. 'I'll have to take this.' He left the room, pulling the door closed behind him.

I waited, feeling increasingly nervous and catatonic. As the minutes ticked by on the clock on the mantelpiece, I could hear his voice in the hall. Forcing myself to stand, I stared round the room with my hands behind my back, scared to touch anything. I could see a paperback book sticking out an angle from beneath files, it was a garish paperback. I peered at the spine. Why on earth did he have a book by Georgette Heyer? Suddenly the door opened and Alexander appeared.
'I just had cramp,' I gabbled, moving back to the armchair.
The room felt too small to have us both standing in and the temptation to touch him was almost overwhelming.
'Sorry about that Undine, a patient being a bit silly and rather insulting. I think rudeness is inexcusable, don't you?'
'Yes,' I said obediently, flattered that he didn't view me in the same light as them. Alex smiled at me warmly.
'Ah, I see you've spotted my secret vice, Georgette Heyer writes very well, I think. Have you read any of hers?'
I hadn't since I was 13 years old; I said this and received an arctic stare.
'Next week, I want homework done Undine, or I really don't think there's much point with us going on.' Alex looked quickly at his watch and ushered me to the door.

Outside, with a sinking feeling, I forced myself to look at a church clock. As I suspected, it was ten minutes before we were due to finish. I would have to try and assert myself at the next session with Alexander and say that I wanted the time added on.

****

Einstein Road

The wooden chair scraped against the floor as Bubbles dragged it back from the kitchen table at Einstein Road. She sat down, carefully blowing crumbs away across the table surface before opening Marius's new notebook, which she'd purloined from beside the bed. The first page was as luminous as virgin snow with delicate lines like blue veins. Bubbles reached for the sharp fountain pen:
'SHE YEARNED FOR LOVE' she wrote in black block capitals, and underlined it carefully using the handle of the bread knife. It was time to buckle down and prostitute her art.

After some thought and a lot of breaks to make cups of tea, Bubbles wrote the following with a view to sending it eventually to Moon & Bonk publishing.

'Ursula, you don't mind keeping an eye on things do you?' Sarah wheedled, already reaching for her jacket.
Ursula smiled and shook her head; her long silky blond hair slid from the neat chignon at the nape of her neck. 'Oh' she reached up quickly, pushing her hair back into the tight roll. 'It suits you, leave it' admonished Sarah. 'No' said Ursula firmly. When she wore her hair loose, people assumed she was sixteen, rather than her 24 years. Sarah said enviously, not for the first time: 'You are lucky you know, size 10, you can wear anything with that tiny waist. There's no justice.' This was an allusion to Ursula's ability to eat anything and not put on an ounce. Ursula knew if Sarah didn't go soon, she would be putting pressure on her again to dress more youthfully. Naturally shy, she preferred to avoid attention by wearing sedate blouses and skirts.

'I won't be long' said Sarah happily, pushing open the ornate glass door, so that the hubbub of Kensington High Street suddenly drowned her words. 'Take as long as you like' said Ursula peaceably, knowing Sarah would lose all track of time once she was at lunch with her friends at Luigi's. Anyway she enjoyed being in charge of Clouds, while Sarah avoided her managerial responsibilities.

*Sarah suddenly halted, letting the door swing closed again.
'Oh Ursula, I'm sorry, I forgot to say: my cousin Anthony has
just taken over Clouds and the other two shops. He's
obviously adding to his empire'. This last was said
sarcastically. She met Ursula's startled green eyes, and
laughed. 'It's OK, he won't bother with us, we're small
compared to his racehorses and other stuff. Anyway the
boutique is doing really well.'
'But you told me he's well, formidable. You remember, when
you asked him if I could rent his flat,' stuttered Ursula. Sarah
had purloined one of her cousin's many assets for her friend.
'Won't he want to visit the shop to check?'
'Oh sometime I expect. He is a bit of a stickler, but he's
bound to ring first' Sarah said reassuringly. With that she was
gone, dark hair flying, Armani suit vanishing into the crowds of
tourists outside.
Ursula walked to the back of the shop, her low court shoes
sinking into the thick carpet. She began to unwrap a new
delivery of dresses, caressing the expensive materials. The
heavily-sequined designer cocktail dress ordered for Mrs
Huysmen had arrived. She was laying it out carefully across
a cream leather sofa in the changing room, when she heard
the shop door open.*

*Ursula emerged to see a very handsome man in an
expensive suit walking across to one of the rails lining the
walls. 'Can I help you?' she asked pleasantly as he began
riffling through the display with long sun-tanned fingers, rather
disparagingly she thought.
He glanced down at her: 'Is Sarah Kendall here?' he asked,
light blue eyes flicking over her dismissively. Ursula found
herself nervously pushing back stray strands of hair.
'Um, no she's meeting a business client for lunch' she heard
herself lying. 'Would you like to leave her a message?' Her
voice trailed off as he strolled past her, still looking at the
clothes.
'Who are you?' he asked arrogantly.
'I'm Ursula Walker, her assistant manager. Would you mind
telling me who you are?' Heavens, why was she being so
rude? As Ursula blushed, he turned and looked down at her
less grimly. 'Not in the slightest' he said: 'I'm Anthony.'
'Oh,' said Ursula startled.*

'Yes, "Oh". Now would you mind telling me where my flighty cousin really is, Ursula Walker? I'd be very surprised if she's at lunch at' he consulted a Rolex wristwatch, '10.35.'
'Well, she is' blurted Ursula loyally, trying to avoid a row. Anthony raised an eyebrow, but let this pass. He pushed a hand through dark hair which showed a tendency to fall across one eye.
'Would you mind showing me the books, and perhaps you could get me a coffee? Black, no sugar.' White teeth flashed in a charming smile.
'Yes of course' said Ursula seething. 'Most of the sales are already on the computer, but here's the receipt book too.' She banged it down on the marble-topped table rather harder than she had intended and marched towards the staff area at the back of the shop to make coffee. If Anthony thought he could patronise her, then charm his way out of it, he was wrong. Amused by this unusual display of temper, Anthony watched Ursula's slender, curvaceous figure disappear behind the curtain veiling the small rest area. His eyes narrowed at the strands of long golden hair falling down her back. A pity she wore such dowdy clothing, plus it didn't reflect well on Clouds. Well it wasn't his problem, her services wouldn't be required much longer. It was time that Sarah earned her own living, instead of frivolously gadding about.

 Ursula was startled to discover Anthony just outside the curtain when she emerged with the coffee in a white and gold china cup, with a biscuit neatly placed in the saucer.
He looked into changing room at the dress draped across the sofa. 'That's for Miss Huysman, she'll collect it later' Ursula explained in response to his enquiring look. She followed him in as he went to examine the price tag. At that moment the shop door opened;
'Oh excuse me,' Ursula pushed the cup of coffee at Anthony. To her horror, he turned too late and the contents fell in slow motion, it seemed, all over the pale dress. Her flustered apologies fell into a dreadful silence. 'I'll pay for the dress' Ursula finished, almost in tears.
'Unless my cousin is paying you far too much, I doubt if you could afford it. Hadn't you better go and see who that is?' asked Anthony coldly, turning away.

'Good morning Miss Huysman,' Ursula greeted her. Her heart sank. Miss Huysman smiled coolly. 'Has my dress arrived, only I wanted to wear it this evening?'

'I'm terribly sorry but it's not quite ready' said Ursula unhappily. Miss Huysman's green eyes lost their artificial warmth immediately. She tossed back glossy auburn hair; 'But you promised it would be ready this afternoon' she said icily.

'And so it would have been Celia, but Miss Walker here has just spilt coffee over it' said Anthony silkily from behind Ursula.

'Anthony!' Celia's cry was of real delight. 'I didn't know you were in town.'

'Well, I've just come to sort out Clouds and my errant cousin' said Anthony smoothly.

'Oh yes, Sarah, well she isn't here much...' agreed Celia, as Ursula moved away towards the rest room. Listening to them catching up on social acquaintances, Ursula suddenly decided she'd had enough. Through a mist of tears she struggled into her coat. She sank down onto a chair for a moment, pulling her shoe on more securely. The bell sounded faintly as the door of the boutique closed. Silence fell.

'Leaving so soon?' the curtain was pulled back abruptly. Ursula looked up startled.

'Yes' she said, suddenly furious. 'How dare you speak to a customer about me like that! I'm leaving-'

'Oh no you're not Miss Walker, you're fired.' he interrupted icily. Here are a month's wages.' He dropped a sealed envelope contemptuously into her open bag.

Ursula rose bravely from the chair, grabbing at her shoulder bag. Cheeks flaming, she had to pass close to Anthony as he didn't move aside. To her dismay, she felt a strand of her long hair snag on one of his jacket buttons. Ursula desperately tugged at the hair - to no avail. She stared at the wall as Anthony freed her, taking his time. As the silky hair slid between his fingers he looked interestedly at her averted profile. She was certainly attractive, flushed like this.

'Thank you' Ursula whispered. She rushed to the entrance and pulled at the heavy glass door. To her intense relief she found herself out in the street, anonymous amongst the

*crowds. That rude, horrible man! How dared he treat her like
that? Ursula's anger turned to anxiety. How on earth was
she to manage without a job? She wouldn't be able to send
her parents money now next month, which she knew they
relied on. She walked numbly towards High Street
Kensington tube station.*

Bubbles heard a key being inserted into the front door and
reluctantly returned to Einstein Road, closing the exercise
book. Laying the pen carefully on the kitchen table, she
shook her hand to ease cramp. Chloris appeared in the
kitchen doorway.
'Hello Undine,' she said loudly, with an artificial smile. She
placed a couple of rustling plastic carrier bags from a
delicatessen beside the cooker and straightened up, lifting her
long hair off her neck with white hands.
'How's the job going? You know you've still got some gold
paint on - just here?' She touched Bubbles' face. Bubbles
recoiled irritably.
'Fine.'
Chloris bent down and began lifting items out of the bags.
Bubbles slid the pen between the pages of her notebook.
'Umm Undine, you know that box of diaries of yours, you keep
in the back room?' Bubbles saw with interest that Chloris
looked embarrassed.
'Yes,'
'Well, I think you should get rid of them.'
'Why?'
There was a brief silence. Chloris bustled around, slapping
food loudly onto shelves inside the unlit 'fridge, her back to
Bubbles.
'This bulb's gone again!'
'Have you been reading them?' Bubbles was intrigued rather
than angry.
'Well, no, but - well I should throw them out. Rosalie,
Matilda's friend, seems to be sleeping in there now.' Chloris
clicked her tongue disapprovingly. 'Do you want me to do it
for you?'
'No! They're just diaries from when I was a child, well the
ones since I was a teenager are fuller...'

Bubbles padded quietly out of the kitchen along the hall towards the back of the house. A damp chill rose from the floor as she drew near to the spare room. Her cardboard box of tatty diaries, of varying sizes, with different years printed on the front covers in tarnished lettering, lay on the black and orange tiled floor outside the closed door. She hadn't ever re-read the diaries. During teenage years and her early twenties they had often been a cathartic out-pouring of anxiety, a waste product of torment. She reached down through them, pushing them aside until she pulled out a small red diary at random and slowly opened it.

Bubbles remembered the threats, as she reluctantly turned the pages with fascinated fear: 'If you ever come home pregnant you'll be out on the doorstep. Get married first.' Grania warning viciously. When I thought about it, I couldn't understand what was wrong with having an illegitimate baby. 'And if you ever end up with a sexual disease, it is a fate worse than death, and you'll go mad and die.' We didn't have a television, computer, or in fact many links at all with a more liberal-minded, contemporary world.

My friend and enemy Woodsy was approved of by parents, always seen as such a nice girl. Only I know she douched herself with her Dad's whisky when she was 15, when the condom came off inside her while she and Andrew were having sex in her parent's bed one afternoon. Her mum and dad were out shopping for a foot spa.

When I thought I might be pregnant I hadn't even had sex, but I was so worried that I had, it being a very bad year with OCD when I was 13, I locked myself in the bathroom and carefully put a knitting needle up there as far as I could to try and get rid of any baby. I'd read in books that that's what people did, or jumped off tables. So I kept leaping off high tree branches and doing gymnastics across the lawn. I couldn't drink gin (my Dad and Grania being teetotal) or get to a clinic and I didn't have the money for a pregnancy test. When I started having sex at 15 I was astonished by how physical it was, there was no mistaking what you were up to. I'd thought before that that you floated off on a romantic pastel cloud of bliss. In the event I was deeply thankful that my face didn't turn bright green or something, so that Grania and my Dad would know what I'd been up to.

Bubbles curiously read the flamboyantly-pencilled prose on a yellowing sheet of paper:
Darling,
I love you so much that the Earth could turn upon the solid axis of it. So much love that birds soar through the liquid skies upon it; that currents of passion propel the rivers; that only because of you, do I understand what the word 'love' means.
She couldn't remember who it was about.

She turned the page:
This is mine, this minute in a music-breathing atmosphere of a small light airy (cold) room just off the Iffley Road. There's a dumb waiter in a cupboard in the corner, a tiny sink, a Baby Belling cooker, a huge chipped oak wardrobe I use as a larder. I've laid it on the side so that it's harder to get food out of. There's a single bed, the springs of which almost touch the floorboards. The landlord, Letchy Stover, is furious and discomfited by the fact that I've dragged the garish nylon carpet and old lino out and dumped them beside the dustbins.

8st 2lbs (not great) but was up to 11stone 3lbs (!) Now 7st 8lbs (legs still fat?) since November.

Bubbles dropped the sheet and it spiralled gently downward, sucked back into the box.

****

Gabriel

This morning, Gabriel had been woken early by the passage overhead of Canada Geese – which made a change from 'planes on the flight path to Heathrow. The birds passed low and honking loudly, large 'Vs' with extended necks, disappearing romantically into the mist. Hermione Puckers, a local bigwig, said they were the devil. Goodies were ducks and moorhens apparently, but Gabriel thought Hermione should remember that there was such a thing as reincarnation.

There was a thump now as the postman threw everyone else's post onto the wooden bench outside the front door. *The Ark* rocked gently as a speedboat zipped past out in the middle of the Thames, the driver blithely ignoring the red 'Slow Down' signs on posts on the outskirts of the small pontoon. Gabriel liked watching the cormorants standing on top of the piles and spreading their wings to dry. When they fished, they dived underneath the water against the fast brown current and, just as he was convinced they were drowning and mentally gulped air, they emerged a long distance upstream with huge fish in their beaks. They tossed these into the air and miraculously engorged them whole down long thin necks.

This had been his home now for four months; Gabriel still awoke experiencing wonderment that he lived in such rural surroundings for a London suburb, and relief that he was not still dossing down in the Cumbrian commune. He had enthusiastically espoused the cause, and found the countryside beautiful, but he needed more privacy, plus warmer, dryer weather. It beat him how anyone retained features let alone grew a beard in west Lancashire, with the wind howling in off the Irish Sea. He'd gone up there partly to do some research for an acting part he'd heard was in the pipeline for the BBC, but which hadn't materialised. By the time he left, cliques were forming. People had begun labelling their milk, or if their benefits hadn't come through, hanging around the cows.

The Ark, bought with the proceeds of his part in a surprisingly successful sitcom, was composed of a Pre-Fab - although it was Fab, even Post-Fab, Gabriel surmised. They'd probably have PhDs on that next. It was a house with six-inch thick timbered walls stuck to a voluminous, one centimetre thick, steel hull. The latter had been used as a barrier to stop boats bumping into the bank - still was, come to think of it, when some stupid arse from a Rowing Club came too close - and as a berth for destroyers during the Second World War. Built to last in fact, except that Gabriel had recently discovered that it might perish due to modern sensibilities, which demanded that the Thames be a picturesque place. Sensible Alison, with the gorgeous behind, who'd sold him the boat, said it had been idyllic on the water before they had erected the exclusive development on the bank, of poky neo-historical flats. Prior to that, there had been a boatyard, a small house and other desirable things such as grass, butterflies and stinging nettles, whilst on the river the same boats had been bobbing up and down for the past twenty years. They were all considerably more picturesque and better-maintained than The [Post-Fab] Ark.

Now, on the bank there were Raybans, Porsches, porches, laptops, boxy modern flats, mobile 'phones, celebrities, new mountain bikes, turf, roundabouts, pristine Landrovers, 'Cyclists Dismount' and 'No skateboarding' signs, Tuscan sun-tans and Chiswick Brayers relaying property prices. Apparently £250,000 was being spent at present renovating the Trust House, and three male Life Guards were going to move in once it was finished. Ali, Kate and Florence, the women on the pontoon, were in a pleasurable state of anticipation.

Gabriel had been told by his neighbour, Dan, who lived next door on a trawler that looked like the sort of jolly boat that children draw, that the eight boats had previously been moored to a wall a hundred yards further along, admittedly with chemical toilets instead of mains drainage. It would have been worth it not to feel as though you resided in a goldfish bowl, Gabriel considered. Passing populace, of which there were thousands nowadays, draped themselves over the pier railings on land and commented on his activities on deck. As he was usually cleaning out the cat litter tray in his jeans before having a shower – they were also Torquil's cats, but he'd managed to make maintaining geraniums in the window boxes his priority – the conversations followed a set pattern. 'Oh look, what sweet cats.' Amazing how exotic domestic animals appear when lazing on a boat deck.
'Puss, puss, puss …' Leo promptly sat down and washed his rear end.
The two women switched their attention to the *homo sapien*. 'What's he doing?'

'I don't know ... [*Appreciative stares at his bare torso.*] Is that a cat litter tray?'
'Oh.'
'I don't think I fancy that *pain au chocolat* now.'

Maybe he'd apply for one of the moorings further out into the river, away from the bank. Some London kids on one of the educational school trips to bring them closer to the river – Gabriel wondered why they didn't just chuck them in – yelled down at him to weed the boat, when *The Ark* was resting on the mud at low tide. Gabriel couldn't summon a cutting rejoinder as there was a purple Buddlia bush sprouting out of the rotting buffer below the bedroom window, not to mention a luxuriant fern beneath the sewage overflow pipe. Now he watched a real seagull's feather float down and conceal an imitation bird, made horribly of dyed feathers, with which Torquil had adorned a Pansy-filled flowerpot.

Torquil hadn't wasted any time upon Gabriel's return to London, approving the boat and declaring himself, temporarily of course, in need of a home. Torquil carried his toothbrush around in his pocket, ever the optimist. Gabriel had met him when he was 22, after moving up to London from Cambridge University to attend RADA – and been dogged by him ever since. When he was travelling and checking out the remains of kibbutz life in Israel, Torquil had written to him daily. Gabriel was relieved not to be one of Torquil's lovers, he suspected they were horrendously harassed. As it was he enjoyed Torquil's witty missives, even the one enclosing a black and white photo he'd taken of a real heart on a plate with a large nail bashed into it (Gabriel hoped it was an animal's) following Torquil's rejection by Dick. He'd read the letters amongst the smell of pines or the squalor of the 'Volunteer House' on a kibbutz near the Golan Heights. Months later he returned in trepidation to Britain, hitch-hiking through Europe for a week on the way with Neil, delaying reaching London. Neil was looking forward to reaching Carlisle, Gabriel had wanderlust and wanted to stay on the road, living on their wits and bravado.

However, climbing off the ferry on to the Sceptred Isle, walking along the mild rain-washed country lanes and seeing small enamelled road signs screwed to stone walls, he had rejoiced. Neil was the one now sad and downcast, and worried that his Dad would find out about their short incarceration in a Dutch prison for vagrancy (insolvency) and ensuing fine. They hitched onwards to the North Circular and the cheap 1950s flat Gabriel had rented previously. He had shared it with Sebastian and a persistent girl from whom he had escaped months before. She was still there, like a protagonist from De Beauvoir's 'She Came to Stay': in fact Sheila opened the flimsy front door to them. Gabriel flinched despite himself. The courtyard below was unkempt and overgrown in the gentle sunlight, which also blessedly illuminated Bella, the tethered malevolent goat. Sheila said accusingly: 'Torquil rang last night, he wondered when you'd be back.'

Gabriel wandered into the tiny kitchen, it felt great to be back amongst friends in familiar surroundings. He and Neil told of meeting Ingrid de Kok and her pimp boyfriend, Guillaume, in a bar, then sleeping in their sitting room back to back because they hadn't trusted the pimp, who was a bastard from hell and who'd slapped Ingrid across the face one evening. Gabriel and Neil had looked so shocked and angry that it had stopped Guillaume in his tracks. Ingrid was kind, blonde and opulently buxom, a stoutly-built glamour puss, who loved and wanted to marry the pimp and live in New Zealand in a little house with frilly curtains and a garden. She carried a dainty hammer with which to tap any troublesome clients who entered her window in the red light district. Gabriel had prayed she'd come to her senses and use it on Guillaume.

'Torquil's been calling a lot, wondering if you're back,' said Sebastian. 'He's a bit persistent isn't he?'

'Can be. Hey, I've got some wine here.' Gabriel unzipped his battered backpack. 'That looks like Torquil's writing, are you two an item?' asked Sheila pruriently. She pointed at a couple of exposed envelopes inside the rucksack.

'No,' he said hurriedly, re-zipping the bag. 'In Torquil's dreams!' said Sebastian laughing. Gabriel changed the subject. There were new carpet tiles on the kitchen floor, but the washing machine he'd rescued from Barnet tip still, endearingly, had its hose tied to the hot tap with a piece of string. Someone, probably Phoebe, had kept the kitchen clean and tidy. 'You can have your old room back if you need it mate,' said Sebastian, his blond corkscrew hair dusty with motes of sunlight. Bella bleated distantly. The telephone rang loudly as Phoebe handed round cups of tea. Sebastian appeared in the doorway to the hall, 'Torquil, for you, Gabriel. Must be telepathic!'

Victor, his agent, hadn't rung so today Gabriel was aboard *The Ark*. He was kept anchored to reality: chores this morning having included washing-up in the bath because the kitchen sink was leaking again. He'd better buy some sealant and have another go at repairing it. Sheila, during their brief liaison, had been used to paying a beautician, Zelda, in Golders Green to have her skin exfoliated. Gabriel considered hiring out the bath now for the purpose, so much of the enamel had worn off. The first time he'd used it he hadn't been able to sit down for days. Gabriel sighed and donned gauntlets, preparatory to applying flea-powder to Camberwell.

Camberwell was one of a shifting population of rescued cats, easily the most intelligent, and the only one not an ardent hunter, choosing instead to supplement his diet of tinned cat food with avocadoes. So when a silver, desperately twirling, eel had appeared beside the sofa a couple of evenings before, he'd ignored it. While Torquil locked himself in the bathroom, Gabriel opened the front door, fingers tingling with fright, hoping the eel would leave in a civilised manner. Leo, another cat, who resembled a large pom-pom, had retaliated to the deprivation of his new toy by being quietly sick on the bath mat. Gabriel only realised this the following morning, stepping out of the shower already late for an audition.

The other cats, Gin and Tonic, were hulking eunuchs. Gin had been called 'Djin', but Torquil's Spiritual Period had been short-lived: he was now entering his Hedonistic Phase. Gabriel just hoped that the duck, Abigail, which apparently nested on deck every year, would have the sense to find alternative accommodation: possibly Denmark. 'Kain' and 'Abel' would have been more suitable names as G&T loathed each other, but they were an invincible team when hunting. During the dawn chorus, they invariably began yelling that they'd caught something, and were dismembering it right outside the bedroom door. If Gabriel forgot, stumbling out blearily to make coffee, chances were that he'd put a bare foot in spongy entrails, or be pierced by a beak lying around in the hall. A white Moroccan rug had had to be hidden, as the cats, united in their admiration of Jackson Pollock, made a point of massacring wildlife on it.

Gabriel had been surprisingly upset when Torquil had taken G&T to France with him: Torquil's love affair with Pierre had made 'Last Tango in Paris' look very tame. Torquil had emigrated in an old ice-cream van, complete with flowered curtains and pastel stripes sprayed on the sides. The chimes of 'Greensleaves' had, eventually, mercifully faded into the din of traffic on the Hogarth roundabout. Unfortunately, he'd reappeared with the cats three weeks later, smuggled through Dover with the van chimes at maximum volume to drown the caterwauling. He arrived just as Gabriel was interviewing a sane and cheerful potential boat-sharer. With regret, Gabriel waved Ian good-bye as Torquil broodingly rearranged the cutlery drawer.

Apparently Gin & Tonic had fitted into the hunting lifestyle of rural France far better than Torquil, bagging plenty of prey. However he had felt it to be his duty to bring them back to London, as he was terrified they'd be shot by equally ardent French hunters, mistaking the rustle in the undergrowth for wild boar. As he wouldn't eat *fois gras*, Torquil stated righteously, he certainly wasn't going to partake of cat paté. It gradually emerged that Torquil had roared off in high dudgeon on two wheels because Kevin had demanded a *ménage a trios,* which French phrase even Torquil comprehended - and with a *femme*! *Quelle horreur.* Gabriel escaped with relief to his local pub, the *George & Devonshire*, for a pint of London Pride with Dan.

On Gabriel's penultimate day in Cumbria, he'd rescued Leo from a farmer, about to drown him in a horse trough. Leopold Bloom had been pretentiously named due to his odyssey from Lancaster to London and had ungratefully defecated in the cat box just as the congested Intercity train sighed in. Gabriel clambered aboard, thankfully finding a seat opposite a small

boy and his mother. For a kitten five inches long, Leo made
an incredible amount of noise during the four-hour journey.
'Mummy, pussy cat don't like box. He's smelly int ee?' Junior
intoned observantly at ten-minute intervals while his mother
tried to distract him, glared at Gabriel and breathed through
her mouth.
'We apologise for the delay, due to engineering works. Our
next station stop will be Warrington Bank Quay, wait until the
train has pulled into the platform stop before disboarding.'
Why did they have to use such appalling grammar on top of
everything else, Gabriel wondered. Part of the infuriating
current drive to obfuscate the meaning of the English
language, no doubt-
'Do we have to discuss your boxer shorts now, Robert?'
'Mum, they've got the The Incredibles on, look!'
'Don't wave them around.'
'He's naughty isn't he Mum?'
'Robert! I won't tell you again. Lyndsey, what are you eating?'
'Nothing.'
'What've you got in thur Mister?' Robert was suddenly
standing in the aisle, staring hungrily at the box and picking
his nose.
'A kitten, Stupid.' Lyndsay prodded Leo's paw waving
through one of the air holes.
The paw disappeared hurriedly.
'Why?'
Leo mewed aggrievedly.
'Pshaw, he stinks.'
'Let's see him.'
'Best not to let him out.'
'Why not?'
Wail of agreement from Leo.
Torquil, who'd had to be bribed into collecting Gabriel from
Euston because of driving across London in the rushhour,
beamed besottedly when Gabriel placed Leo on his palm.
Leo pungently and devotedly stared back. Gabriel had
already discovered that Leo (surprisingly) liked men, so he
and Torquil had that in common. Also that Leo could fart tear-
gas.

Being a floating animal rescue centre, though he was
uncertain what species Torquil was, had involved sacrifice on

Gabriel's part. He had given up inviting potential girlfriends to dinner since the Charlie debacle. He seemed to be fatally attracted to women who left half-way through the evening, wheezing and streaming. During through the starter, Sarah had said accusingly, Charlie's *so* allergic to cats. Charlotte had nodded vehemently from behind a handful of tissues. 'Now Jake that's *so* not true, it is cats. She hasn't used coke for ages, not since that job in the City, have you Chas?' The tissues shook furiously.

Charlotte emerged, red-eyed: 'Sorry, I should be all right, Gabriel, so long as I don't actually *touch* a cat.' Charlotte smiled apologetically at Gabriel whose heart leapt, and slid sinuously into her seat next to him at the supper table. During dessert, Leo leapt on to Charlotte's lap like a bouncing bomb, whereupon she was whizzed efficiently off to Casualty by Benedict in his Ferrari. Charlie waving with the hand not holding tissues, still managing to look frail and beautiful with streaming eyes and an atomiser sticking out of her nose. Next thing Gabriel knew, Charlotte and Benedict were advertising their wedding banns in 'The Times'.

Camberwell had ear mites again; Gabriel reflected that taking the cats to the vet on the bus was enough to make him take up smoking. He had sustained bloody scratches around the ears unsuccessfully trying to lure a vindictive Camberwell into the cat-box last time. Gin would submit to being shoved in backwards, while vociferously complaining, like a Sloane into a Council flat. Camberwell promptly bonded with Torquil, hanging from his shoulders at meal-time like an exotic wrap, grabbing food from Torquil's fork as it approached his mouth, both of them glancing smugly at Gabriel. At night Camberwell purred loudly on the other pillow and braced cold paws against Gabriel's face. When he ruefully surveyed his photo in last year's 'Spotlight', one without bags under his eyes and scratch marks, and dared to mention the fact that Gin was sitting on his computer keyboard scratching again, Torquil inferred he was an old fart. When he shut the cats out of the bedroom at night, G&T tried to tunnel under the door with Leo hissing encouragement.

****

Bubbles

Back at Einstein Road, Bubbles ran quietly upstairs two at a time and threw her bag into her room. She returned more slowly to the kitchen and peered in. To her great relief the room was sunlit and empty, and the washing-up had been done. Sometimes she did Chloris's housework, even though she herself didn't cook, because she was so repulsed by the grubby work surfaces and grease-splashed cooker.

Bubbles opened her exercise book and unscrewed the top of her fountain pen. She put the bottle of ink carefully to one side. She turned to a clean page in her book and pressed it flat:

Sarah said crossly: 'Ursula's a really good worker. She gets on well with all the customers, in fact lots of them come back just to see her. It would have to be Celia's dress which was spoilt.' Her tone showed her low opinion of Celia Huysman. Anthony tried to excuse himself: 'Well that dress was £1,200 and it's ruined. And you have to admit Ursula dresses as though she's fifty - not a very good advertisement for Clouds.' Sarah ignored this: 'It sounds as though Celia's dress was partly your fault' said she accusingly. 'Ursula's usually very careful'.
Sarah 'phoned Ursula that evening, but heard only the answerphone. She left an apology for her cousin's behaviour, furiously thinking Anthony should be the one contacting her friend, and offering Ursula her job back.

Sarah's annoyance increased during the next three weeks. Anthony often visited the shop, which forced her to remain at Clouds, apart from official breaks for lunch or coffee. Used to a far more leisurely existence, Sarah finally snapped at her troublesome cousin that profit wasn't everything. Irritated, Anthony ungraciously conceded defeat. If Sarah must, she could offer Ursula her job back. But although she continued to phone, Sarah only heard Ursula's pleasant answerphone message. She felt hurt when Ursula didn't return her calls, and began to feel anxious. She hoped her friend was just taking time to get over Anthony's high-handedness and had found another job.

Ursula had not found something else; she had been to the Job Centre and was looking dutifully in newspapers, but nothing had turned up. She was too humiliated and proud to accept Sarah's telephone protestations that she could have her old job back. 'I'm not accepting charity from Anthony' she thought furiously, tossing and turning during sleepless nights. She guessed that her friend must have pestered her obnoxious cousin into relenting. Ursula was becoming worried about money - and also the fact that the flat belonged to Anthony. Did he realise who was renting it? Ursula no longer wanted to live there; all the pleasure had gone out of her attractive home. One night she found herself worrying about small repairs that needed doing; the doorbell hadn't worked properly in ages, the bath tap dripped, the letter-box was so stiff that the postman obligingly left her mail outside the door or with her neighbour. Would Anthony charge her? She wouldn't put it past him to turn up and evict her. Oh, for heaven's sake Ursula, she thought, stop this! She plumped up the pillow again and tried to sleep.

'I don't want to live here any more anyway' she said bravely aloud, as she cooked for herself the following evening. Ursula was aware this wasn't true, and pulled a rueful face as she stirred the pasta. She couldn't raise the huge deposit necessary for an equally attractive flat in London. She sighed, and decided to pamper herself with a scented bath before supper, maybe it would make her feel better.

Emerging refreshed and happier, Ursula towelled her long hair as dry as possible, then wrapped herself in a large white fluffy towel. She paused as she thought she heard a noise, but decided it was the bathroom fan. She padded into the hall. Seeing a movement in the hall mirror, Ursula spun round to see the front door slowly opening. Frozen to the spot, she opened her mouth to scream as a tall figure moved slowly forward into the shadowy hall.
'Oh, I am sorry, I rang several times but no-one answered' said Anthony smoothly. His eyes narrowed as he looked down at her. Ursula felt herself trembling with delayed shock. 'What are you doing here? I was having a bath!' she blurted out.

'Yes, I can see that, a mermaid,' he said softly. His eyes moved appreciatively down to her toes showing beneath the towel, then back to her blushing face. Her heart thumped. Defensively, Ursula tried to push her damp hair back over her shoulders, then to her horror felt the towel sliding apart at the back. She began to back towards the bedroom.
'Could you wait in the sitting-room please?' she asked sternly.
'Certainly, Ursula Walker,' he said, smiling.

Hurriedly closing the bedroom door behind her, Ursula sank onto the bed, then leapt up and began shakily climbing as fast as possible into loose jeans and a sensible short-sleeved top. She draped a towel across her shoulders and spread her hair across it to dry. She stared into the mirror seeing wide pale green eyes, fringed by dark lashes. Her long blonde hair, still damp, hung down in long tresses. No wonder he'd likened her to a mermaid.
As Ursula came out of the bedroom she glanced towards the hall mirror - and froze. Anthony had laughed as she ordered him into the sitting room - because he could see the slipping towel reflected in the mirror as she backed away. What else had he seen? A wave of warmth swept her from head to foot. Outside the sitting room door, she tried to breathe evenly, but her heart hammered.

Anthony was lying lazily in the armchair facing the door. He flicked back his glossy hair and rose to his feet as she came in.
'A pity' he commented, surveying her unflattering clothes. A faint line of irritation appeared between his dark brows.
'How I dress is my affair! And I would like to know why you're here, invading my privacy. The least you could do is to apologise'. Usually polite and considerate, Ursula was newly astonished by her hostile response. But it was unforgivable that he had entered the flat. She was also uneasily aware that she had to remain on her guard against Anthony. The treacherous feelings of weakness he aroused in her when they met, meant she might easily become another of his conquests.
'I have apologised' he pointed out gently; he smiled at her and her heart lurched at the warmth in his gaze. 'Sarah's worried because she hasn't been able to get you on the 'phone. Your

*letter-box doesn't work either, or I would have pushed this
letter through.'*
*'No, I've been meaning to ask about fitting a new letter-box
…'. It was a relief to be talking about something so mundane.
'I actually came here, under pressure it must be admitted, to
offer you your job back' he said carefully, standing up.
Ursula felt a stab of anger at the words "under pressure". It
was as she'd suspected, Sarah had forced him into it.
'Thank you, but I don't want the job,' she said icily.
'Thank you for the "thank you",' Anthony mocked, pushing his
hands into his pockets and rocking on his heels slightly. 'Is
that a "No" then?' he asked disbelievingly.
'Yes' she said stiffly. 'I don't suppose you want a cup of
coffee do you?'
Anthony laughed outright. He said wickedly, 'I would love a
cup of coffee, although I get the feeling you'd like me to go.'
'Not at all' she muttered untruthfully, hurrying through the
swing door into the small kitchen. Ursula let out a groan and
hurriedly turned off the cooker. She rushed to open the
window to let out the smell of burnt pasta.
'Oh dear' said Anthony sardonically, just behind her.
Ursula turned quickly and found herself looking up at him.
She couldn't think of anything to say. Rather than look at him,
she stared intently at the heavy signet ring on the little finger
of his right hand. It had his initials engraved on it. Ursula
tried to move round him in the confined space, back to the
safety of the sitting-room. When she had trapped herself in a
corner of the kitchen, she saw that he was watching her
intently.
'It's okay, I'm not going to attack you - Ursula' he said smiling.
He turned and held open the door for her. Feeling like an
idiot, Ursula stalked through. He was laughing at her again.
She would not show him the effect his use of her name had
on her. If only he would go-*

Damn, here's Matilda.

Matilda wandered in and smiled at Bubbles, began making a
pot of tea, then padded past the table *en route* to her shelf in
the food cupboard. She stopped.

'Is that a *Mont Blanc*?' She leant her hip against the table and stared down at the pen. Bubbles hurriedly picked it up, replacing the cap. 'I don't know, I found it.'

'Cool. They're really expensive,' Matilda took the pen from Bubbles's fingers and inspected it enviously; Bubbles resisted the temptation to snatch it back.

'It's even a Millenium special, la! Sorry, you really mind me looking at it, don't you?' She stared down at Bubbles with a hint of malice.

'No, of course not,' lied Bubbles.

Matilda dropped the pen negligently back onto the notebook and sauntered on.

'Cup of tea?'

'Oh yes please, I'll just move this stuff.' Bubbles gathered up her writing things and bore them up to her room, placing them neatly on the floor by the bird-cage.

She almost fell downstairs on her way back, walking in a big semi-circle to avoid the ironing board on the landing. Bubbles had bravely chipped off and disposed of the old asbestos on the iron rest (Chloris had wanted to throw the whole board out). Now Bubbles kept washing her hands in case she had some asbestos left on her fingers and transferred it to door-handles, or deliberately poisoned some stranger.

****

Gabriel

I've finally remembered to lower the blind in the kitchen against curious stares from bank-dawdlers ten foot away. This is because last night I woke up hungry and stumbled naked through the dark kitchen to the refrigerator. When I opened the 'fridge door, the light came on and I heard loud inebriated cheers. I slammed the door, but it continued. I peered at the bank and waved angrily out of the window at the whine bar crowd to move on, and they waved back - the cheek of it! Torquil said I should have mooned, *Free Willy* v. *Moonstruck,* but like most sequels it would have been anti-climactic.

Speaking of unintentional exhibitionism, I can't angle the
Venetian blinds in the bathroom effectively due to the
vagaries of the tide, which gives the guy who lives in a
penthouse on the bank something else to complain about.
The residents on *terra firma* regard us as water gypsies,
which is fine by me. Other responses fall neatly into two
categories:
'Oh, I've always wanted to live on a boat!' people say
jealously. The other fifty per cent look horrified and ask if I've
got a toilet. If I dislike them, I just murmer furtively about
buckets, which immediately silences any hints about how
difficult it is to view the Boat Race properly from the bank.

As I now stroke shaving foam onto my face, I remember
Alison warning me against filling the bath too full:
'When the boat rocks, it floods the bathroom, it happened to
me once. Then you've got it all going through the floor down
into the hold, a real nuisance'.
Unfortunately it's already happened once since I moved in,
hence the presence of a humming de-humidifier. Lulled by
the fact that *The Ark* hadn't rocked for a while (it usually
happens when you're standing on a kitchen stool) I'd
forgotten that I was floating in water, on water. I was
fascinated to note surface tension momentarily held the water
on the edge of the bath, then I couldn't get the plug out fast
enough. My glass of red wine and Library book both fell into
the water which made me look like an extra in a Greek
tragedy. Why do nasty things happen in threes? Which
brings me on to the water heater, another potential expense.

'The thermostat's broken, didn't I mention it?' Alison said,
handing over the keys in exchange for a ridiculously large
cheque for a floating shed. She gathered up the dog leads
with a worrying sigh of relief. 'It's all right, as long as you
remember to switch it off before the water boils over from the
tank in the hall' she called merrily, being towed away to
somewhere glorious in Wales by Tom, her Border Collie. I
must remember to stick a note on the cupboard door.

I can hear a politician shrilly defying John Humphries on the
radio: 'We cannot afford the medications for the condition'. I
grimace at myself in the mirror: does everyone have to adopt

the American habit of not knowing the difference between singular and plural? I admit it: I'm an anachronism, a pedant. I find myself shouting at News presenters and others who should know better on Radio 4, for using grammar erroneously, I click my tongue at grammatical errors in the broadsheets and decry the decline of the adverb. Do we all have to speak in journalese? Everything is rushing past so fast, there's no need to accelerate it. It would explain all those unfortunate joggers: perhaps evolutionarily-advanced humans can no longer walk, only run. Criminals could escape easily along the tow-path here, everyone would just think they were training for the London Marathon.

Anyway, no-one knows how to use prepositions correctly any more, and as for the poor apostrophe – I must join that organisation that campaigns for their appropriate use. Apparently a woman who's written a book about the correct use of the apostrophe says her least favourite sentence is: 'Get a life'. I don't care: language is supposed to aid communication, not obscure it! Damn, that would have been an exclamation mark, cheap punctuation, if it had appeared on a printed page.

Narrow sideburns today I think, even if I am entitled to wear the Victorian mutton-chop variety. The razor makes tiny scratching sounds. I'm shattered. The cats and I are currently sleeping on a sofa-bed mattress that's too small for the bed frame. This is causing territorial disputes worthy of the Middle East: it's always me who wakes in the dark, small, hours on the wooden slats. Occasionally a cacophony of snores emanates from the dark hump which is Torquil, lonely and needing my – platonic - company for a night, and rolled up in my duvet like a snail in its shell. Last night Leo misjudged the distance between boat and bank and landed in the mud, luckily the tide was out or he'd have splashed into thirty foot of water. He jumped onto my head – my heart tried to clear my chest - then dripped his way morosely across the clean duvet cover. I was a bit fed-up because I'd only stamped up and down on the bed linen in the bath on Wednesday. The washing machine has yet to be plumbed in and the local laundrette, which is lovely, with flowering pot plants and a friendly dog, is open on a capricious basis. I could hear liquid mud dripping between the slats onto the carpet round the edge of the bed while Leo stood heavily on my stomach, purring as his paws dried out. I nudged Torquil, then pretended to be asleep. Torquil awoke, switched on the light, screeched disapprovingly, then I could feel him looking at me suspiciously. Mind you, despite being a *hausfrau extraordinaire,* he draws the line at chipping rejected cat food off the floor. Come to think of it, it has hitherto unexploited adhesive qualities. It might do as cheap glue…

I rinse my face with warm, then cold,water. I toy with the idea of trying out some moisturiser that Torquil's given me, but don't like the smell when I sniff at it experimentally. Finn is supposed to be dropping round a new mattress, I can't wait. Unfortunately Finn being knee-high to a gnome and professionally lazy doesn't facilitate delivery, so I'll have to. He hasn't been able [willing] to lift it into the van on his own, apparently it's a heavy futon. That should correct the list on *The Ark*: the floor slopes quite dramatically at the moment at high tide. Conversely perhaps it's a middle–class mattress and believes in deferred gratification.

****

Bubbles

I can't remember much else from the early therapy sessions; Alexander did sometimes over-run the time on earlier appointments so that I had to wait in the baronial entrance hall, but I didn't mind too much. He occasionally spent longer with me, but I don't recall seeing anyone else waiting. Sometimes I walked around the block, if I felt too scared and trapped indoors. Once a beautiful girl with waist-length dark hair arrived as I was leaving. She was polite and extrovert, standing aside for me with smiling courtesy. A disorientating pang of jealousy accompanied me up the staircase to pavement level.

Sometimes Alexander said things that showed he hadn't listened. He was unreliable regarding booking appointments. He was difficult to contact and seemed to be rushed and disorganised: he forgot to tell me until the last minute when he would be away on holiday. I was thankful that I hadn't told him anything that caused me anxiety about his response. The first two hour-long sessions, I kept blurting out painful pieces of my past, but not the stuff about my brother. Alexander hadn't read all of my form by the third session, and sometimes some of my session time would be spent by him hunting for my file ... Nevertheless, we held the course of treatment together. One day he stammered slightly: it turned out that his speech impediment was so severe when he was a child that he couldn't speak. With me, the inner torment causes me to say things I don't want to, or don't mean.

Actually, I do remember things about the early sessions. It seemed as though I learned important, crucial things almost accidentally, a tangential comment caught in passing, fragments of speech.
'People with OCD are hard on themselves, it's part of the condition,' Alexander murmured quietly one day. This effortlessly seemed to grant me permission to stop agonising about the family stuff; it only lasted for a few weeks but still seemed miraculous. I knew Alex was also training to be a hypnotist: I suggested flippantly that he was hypnotising me, he replied gravely that he wasn't.

Another day, I blurted 'get me a tissue' as tears erupted from my eyes, I then worried that I'd been too abrupt, but he said that I hadn't come across as rude at all and stroked my arm. Had he forgotten that I'd told him I hated people touching me without permission? Perhaps he was doing it to "desensitize" me? I mean, there was nothing sexual about it, not on his side anyway. I keep looking at the firm white flesh on the inside of my arm with wonder. I know how smooth it is because I caress it to try and see how it felt to him, it smells nice too.

Being with Alexander is akin to relaxing in a warm bath, in some ways he must be a born healer. I step off a cliff, treading air with him, but once he's gone I look down and the trouble starts. Between sessions it's hard to manage without the support. Sometimes I start awake in the middle of the night and think incredulously, with embarrassment: *I said that to him?* On one hand, it's peculiar how calming he is, how I seem subconsciously to obtain permission from him to do things. Is it because he's a man? I am slowly beginning to feel more empowered now, one grain of sand at a time. On the other, I still experience this shocking fear of lack of control over the sessions, so that I'm shaking by the time I reach up to press the brass doorbell. Perhaps other therapists would just capitulate and work my way, at my pace? I'm worried that Alex is not going to be willing to do that. I don't think he's a good judge of when I'm up against my limit. I've felt once already that he's trying to push me further, beyond which I feel shell-shocked and distressed. It's frightening and a form of bullying, I should know, I've done it to others.

The other week, he gave an incredulous and critical response to the way I acted towards William and his wife a couple of years ago, which has caused me a lot of anguished rumination. I'm confused: it also doesn't sit well with Alexander's view that people with OCD give themselves a hard time and that we should practice compassion on ourselves.

I've realised something: I keep erecting a Grania-type wall of words to shield myself from too much real communication with Alexander. I'm accepting money from Marius to attend sessions and borrowing Matilda's bicycle, and then wasting sessions telling anecdotes or getting Alexander to talk about himself to stop him getting close. I'm too scared of losing control to let him do his job properly. But I can't tell him the thing that has dominated my life for several years now - especially after his recent reaction - and caused me for at least a year to 'cease to function properly'. English Understatement.

[Alexander made a note in Undine's file: 'UC phobic about pens outside her home.']
I couldn't get her to touch a pen, she stepped backwards. Where the hell's my fountain pen? I've looked everywhere, it's one of my favourite things. Plus it was a present from Lucy and she went ballistic last time. I can't even replace it on the sly, it was one of a limited edition.

****

At Einstein Road, Bubbles pushed the box of diaries back against the wall. She hadn't told Grania or her Dad about the threatening kerb-crawling men, because she was scared of an uncaring response. Some remark about how she deserved it, or convenient deafness. There were a lot of incidents like that: people sense when you are vulnerable and prey on you accordingly. Her rage, feelings of helplessness, inadequacy and fear – it all came out in hating men, despising them, when she moved to London three years later.

It was very hard living for so long isolated in the bedsit. 'What was I just thinking about..?' I had wondered, standing beside the wardrobe.
The answer should have been 'Yes' not 'No', did I say anything aloud? If I said 'No' twice, it means yes, two negatives make a positive.
'Yes' I said in a strangled voice aloud to counter anything I might have said before. Someone's still knocking at my flimsy wooden door. My face feels locked with iron tension, I'm biting my tongue so hard I'm scared I'll bite through it. I have before, at the side. I'm all spotty but if I don't stop squeezing and scrubbing my face I'll never be able to go out again. The

loud banging continues. I open the door a crack. Two of the students, privileged layabouts from downstairs, are there. 'Are you all right?' asks Dave, I think that's his name. He's short and plump, with dark hair and a worried expression. The taller guy says: 'Only we heard you shouting and…' 'Oh yes,' I force my face into a smile, it feels like a rictus ' I'm just practicing for a play I'm in.' They don't look convinced, but slowly walk away, I see Dave look back as I quickly shut the door.

****

Gabriel

It's not good for me lying awake; I've ended up on the bed slats again. Now I've experienced a bit of success being Roger in the sitcom, with money coming in until recently, it's hard to return to being broke and philosophical. I'll have to go and sign up with an agency tomorrow for office work: I'd hoped never to have to do that again. *Oddball Selection* telephone research keep giving the work to other resting actors, they probably see me as 'successful' now. If it weren't for Torquil's trickle of rent I'd be really up against it.

Perhaps my inventions will bring in some money. Yesterday I thought of tiles with ready-trodden-in chewing gum effect: 'Save all that chewing and jaw-ache!' I need someone to promote my ideas, a fusion between inspired creativity and hard cash. Trouble is I can't detach my bike from the railings since Torquil rashly tested my remote-controlled bike lock on it outside Turnham Green Tube. I wonder if the bolt-cutters are in the shed on land.

Torquil's snoring again, I wish he and Pierre hadn't split up. Despite myself I'm beginning to breathe at the same tempo as him. *Ergo:* dramatically inhale, rasping slowly up to a crescendo, becoming louder each time, a click at the summit of the mountain, a worrying silence, then just as I'm going blue around the lips, a long whistling exhalation down a gentle slope. I bet they split up due to Torquil snoring. Now he's bloody well grinding his teeth, just for a bit of variety.

Shit! The hissing noise coming from the hall isn't Leo, but the water tank boiling over.

****

Bubbles

She was five years old and swinging on the high school gate one afternoon when a mother scolded her for scratching her son on his arm. 'Hugh was up all last night with it, it's infected. You're a bad little girl!" she said angrily. The child continued to stand on the bottom bar of the moving gate, uneasily looking at the woman through the black iron railings in wonder and embarrassment. Eventually she awkwardly stepped back and down onto the concrete playground and skipped away.

Childhood and adolescence were about being in a windy, scary, place with nothing solid to hold on to. When Bubbles began learning Physics at 11, the proton/neutron diagram they drew in their exercise books encapsulated the family structure for her: Grania and William bonded closely in the centre, whilst she and her father circled separately, electrons in outer darkness.

Living at 'home' was akin to tip-toeing across a sheet of thin glass. Being painfully honest and her words being denied, or causing people to looking shocked, made her scared to speak. Words were dangerous. Trying to communicate with Grania felt like being punched on a bruise. Grania ignored her, nagged incessantly, or shouted at her.

One of the boys in the village showed her a beautiful grass snake one day, which he kept in his blazer pocket. It was smooth and muscular to stroke. She felt pity for it as he took it out and tied it in knots. It gently tried to right itself, helplessly and uncomprehendingly.

****

Therapy Session

'I had doubts about coming to see a male therapist.'
I meant to sit still today, but already I'm pushing fingers
frenziedly through my hair, raking it back.
Alexander suddenly has that pleased attentive look, which
usually spells a hard session.
'Yes Undine, a lot of female patients say that. Some of them
have issues about men that they can work out here. But me
being a man ultimately doesn't make any difference,'
Bollocks.
'I've had prisoners transferring their mothers onto me.' He
suddenly looked as though he regretted divulging that.
'So you might as well be a chair,' I said lightly.
'Exactly,'
He suddenly looks sad. Unless you've been painted by Van
Gogh, it's probably not a lot of fun being a chair.

I try and tell Alex why I have problems talking on the 'phone,
but half-way through I suddenly realise that I'm probably
mentally ill and how mad the stuff I'm telling him sounds. I
stop abruptly. Alexander says something about 'normalising'
stuff for me; for pity's sake, how ridiculous is that?

Later, when Alexander's calmed me down by speaking
soothingly and stroking my back, I say lightly:
'You remember we talked about the man outside the cinema?
'Er, yes.'
'Well, it really helped.'
'Good.'
'I've even had some fun and not felt guilty!'
'Are you and Marius still together?'
'Yes. I saw this lush man at Camden Lock and instead of
thinking, 'No, don't think that!' and panicking, I just looked at
him. He didn't see me and I walked on. I'd forgotten about
him and I was getting into a bit of state, kept looking back to
make sure I hadn't dropped anything… Anyway, I looked up
and saw him staring at me in exactly the same way that I'd
looked at him earlier. It was like catching a ball in an
important game. I just walked on, I smiled all the way home.
And none of it mattered. It was great.'
'Good, that sounds healthy,' he was smiling.

I made that up, lied, embellished the truth - what you will - and I'm not worried about it. The fact that Alex isn't upset about me fancying someone else hasn't changed my feelings for him one iota. As I leave, he compliments me on my black wide-brimmed hat and long velvet coat. I suppose it would seem dramatic to him, old jean-genie. He should have seen me at that party last year, wearing body paint, with tattoos and gold chains linking my body piercings. It would have blown his tiny mind.

I'm getting a vibe off Undine; she was looking at me during our session this morning, she thought I didn't realise. She's very attractive if you like waifs, she just doesn't press my buttons. I trust her though not to suddenly strip off, like that woman did last year. I was trying to help the patient with her perception of herself as ugly. It was so boring I was almost asleep, I didn't see it coming at all ... One minute she was wearing sensible garb, the next Botticelli's Venus had arrived at Eaton Place. Perhaps she'd Sellotaped her clothes together beforehand. She'd make a brilliant Stripper if she were to slow down a bit, otherwise punters would complain of the blur.
'Can you see anything wrong with this?' she asked me miserably, turning a surprisingly resplendent body. I managed to get out of my seat and behind the chair just in time. I couldn't face an undignified scramble getting her off my lap. I calmed her down from afar and managed to talk her back into her Dannimac. We got some good work done after that session, I think she's a Naturist now.

Since then a couple of colleagues have told me of experiences with patients only able to relate to people sexually. X said that he had a young guy who posed arrogantly, draping himself over the couch and leaving his flies undone during two sessions, until X mildly mentioned his unconventional behaviour. The guy fainted.

Y told me about this middle-aged woman whose voice at each session became higher and younger, and her clothing became trendier, until one day she arrived with her hair tied up in ribbons and wearing a mini skirt. Her body language

was odd: she kept crossing and uncrossing her legs, splayed them apart … At which point he realised with shock that she wasn't wearing any underwear.
'What did you do?' I asked.
'I leaned forward and –' He fell silent.
'What!'
'I said: "I can see your vagina. Do you want to talk about it?" She cried for ages. Then we talked properly for the first time since she's been coming to see me.'

Lucy's my ideal. Calm older women of independent means, if a bit diminished now she's down to a size 18. Probably a mother-complex or something. Good job I'm not a Freudian, ha ha! Yes, I know I have the odd adventure, but you only live once and what the eye doesn't see … Anyway Wendy came on really strong.

****

Bubbles

I really admire Alexander; it must be fascinating being an OCD therapist, seeing a stranger walk towards you and then trying to discover what is at the root of their terrible anxiety and rituals, in order to effect psychological and physiological ease. It must be very difficult if patients don't manifest their problems in rituals, but only ruminate and worry. The therapist would need to have a stable cast of mind, not to become mired in the bog of anxiety and perception of the client. I presume they'd have to have great social skills, or kindness, or ambition for career advancement, prestige or money – or any number of permutations of these - to succeed in not frightening off the sufferer with incomprehension or impatience, and yet be able to enter their world with sufficient empathy to help them. Makes the brain reel really.

****

Einstein Road

'You know, Bubbles is behaving oddly, upstairs.' Matilda said quietly to Chloris. Chloris was making bread, stubby fingers pulling and kneading the pale elastic bread dough. She pushed the door closed with her foot and turned wide blue eyes on Matilda, 'Why, what's she doing?'

'She keeps opening her bedroom door, she's on the landing, peering round it, then pulling it to, not closing it, then doing it all over again.'

'Do you think we should talk to her?'

'I don't know. She looked at me as I passed but she was very pale and strange. She was muttering something too.'

'You know that awful conversation last week, when she kept asking if we thought if she was a coward?'

'Yes, why did she keep asking the same questions, was she not listening or something? It felt as though if I gave the "wrong" answer she might crack up.'

'I know. I almost said, what answer do you want me to give? It reminded me of being at work.'

'It's like living with a stranger. I used to think when I first moved in she hadn't got a care in the world.'

'There's something wrong there. Undine's manic, look at the amount of housework she does. She was washing the wainscoting in the hall early yesterday morning, really scrubbing at it, talking to herself, and I have to go out now when she starts labouring away with that ancient Hoover.'

'It's a bit difficult to do that at seven in the morning. I'm glad I'm at the top of the house, Dion and I can't really hear it up there. Perhaps she's taking too much speed?'

'I'd feel bad if I asked her to leave when she's having a difficult time. I just wish she would pay some rent. Vivienne was really fed-up with her, and Finn, at the last meeting.'

'I know. She owes me too.'

'Oh well,' Chloris added briskly to Matilda's surprise, dropping the dough into a baking tin: 'I like Undine, odd-bod that she is.'

'So do I, you can't help it somehow.'

****

Gabriel

I cycled to Hammersmith along the towpath this morning on Torquil's bicycle (his saddle's a strange shape) feeling like Miss Jean Brodie and wishing I'd taken the time to fetch my expensive bicycle from the shed on the bank instead. I can't use my racing bike as the wheel is bent irredeemably from disentangling the lock I invented, so it's back to the drawing-board. Instead of being able to get up some speed, I was forced to sail serenely aloft with hands either end of the unwieldy handlebars. When I reached the main road, this meant I had as much ability to duck, dive and generally save my life amongst hostile London motorists as a turtle on the M4.

Almost impecunious, I'd finally forced myself to set about enrolling with a Secretarial Agency. Why wasn't *Manpower* called *Personpower*? My Kiwi friend, Kylie, said Temping's a doddle. Come to think of it, she said that about working in that restaurant in Covent Garden three summers ago BR (Before Roger). I made big tips as she'd promised, but it was incredibly hard work, very hot. All the kitchen staff looked like cadavers, they were so pale and knackered. You could see customers thinking they didn't want anything cooked by Tony, who was wearing yesterday's clothes along with last year's bags under his eyes.

I wore my black suit, bought for a funeral, to the agency in the end: not because I subscribe to corporate clothing crap, but because Camberwell who does, ripped my Levis. I was at the spacious blue-carpeted office above the Amusement Arcade for over two hours. I remember this syndrome from a visit to a hospital and the Benefits office, both ages ago now fortunately. They assume that because you're a patient, or unemployed, you have all the time in the world.
Joy, a big-busted, sluttish woman slowly typed the details of my fictional work experience from my form into her computer with long red fingernails. Obviously not speedy enough on the keyboard to procure Temp work, she'd ended up as an interviewer.
'You look familiar, have I met you before?'
'No.' I'm depending on my hair being so much shorter now. I hope she doesn't recognise me from Channel 4, or my CV's down the drain, also it's embarrassing being spotted.
The 'phone rang, saved by the bell.

'No Sam, sorry I've nothing in today.' Joy said, still looking penetratingly at me. She pushed a button. 'I wish she'd stop ringing, I should have put her through to you, Roy.'
'No point, she hasn't got the skills I want. I'm rushed off my feet.' Rob Roy in 'Permanents' flicked at the front of his carrot-coloured hair and leafed importantly through a pile of registration forms.
'Oh, so am I, it's so hectic.' Silence reigned. A large moth fluttered behind the vertical slats of the blind. Joy's bright, cold eyes rested on me.
'Now I need to test you Gary.'
'Gabriel,' I said faintly.
'I'll just key the tests into the computer, it's one for *Excel* isn't it? And this one for *Word* and a little office procedure test, nothing to worry about Gary. Oh and also the spelling test.'

Honestly, the more ill-paid or mundane a job is, the more humiliating the selection procedure: take auditions. But accountants don't have to suddenly do a Bank Reconciliation in two minutes flat, parasitic lawyers do not have to argue a succinct case in under five minutes, or ever. Faced with a three-minute typing test, my keyboard skills evaporate into thick-fingered fumbling. Grip on the keys isn't aided by the fact that they are slippery with the perspiration of previous incumbents. Torquil would have whipped out a disinfected cloth and fastidiously wiped it all down first. The closely-typed pages for copying were all about virtual reality call centres. What a waste of trees, I also saw a couple of grammatical errors. In the panic of the moment I wondered if I should return to paid Waiting in restaurants.

Amazingly, I've landed a three-month Temp job at Hammersmith Hospital, misleadingly named being next to Wormwood Scrubs, location for the 1970s sitcom, *Porridge.* I wish I'd been an actor during the seventies, the golden age of British television comedy. That's my opinion, Torquil swears by US imports like *Frasier.* Rob seemed very reluctant to let me do a PA job for a surgeon, the details of which I could read upside-down on his desk, but indecently keen that I should cover Reception work in the MRI Unit.
'It looks very interesting, you also have to screen visitors for guns,' he said, surveying the job description. I just said, Cool,

nonchalantly. As a pacifist I need to do my bit. I visualised Hammersmith Hospital as being conveniently situated round the corner. Apparently that's Charing Cross Hospital; Hammersmith Hospital is on the 72 bus route or a difficult bike ride. By the time I realised this I was too exhausted to register with another agency, so I spent my last change on a 'Gobbles' Brownie instead. After I'd eaten it I remembered they'd been taken over by heinous McDumps. Still, at least the job might prove useful background for a future medical acting job, think positive, no experience is ever wasted. Speaking of which, there was this girl miming as a gold statue at Hammersmith Mall, when I dropped into Tescos. Hope she's thinking positive. If you drop money into the box at her feet, she moves and hands out vouchers. I wonder if she's an actress, she's really pretty under the paint. I'd like to get to know her, but she's probably allergic to cats too.

I met Kylie for a drink at Café Rogue last night and she was amazed: 'They're paying you that much an hour, to do Reception work? They must be desperate to fill the job. Did I tell you about when I Temped in that hell-hole urinary hospital?'
Yes, often.

****

Bubbles

I wonder what would happen if I told Alexander that he dominates my thoughts?
I am obsessed now by the obsessions expert; but perhaps that's meant to happen. All the obsessive urges move to Alex, then he magicks them away. At this rate though, my compulsive side will triumph and I'll suddenly grab his hand, or worse. Perhaps I'll know the treatment is working when this flood of emotion dries up? I feel possessed. As I try and keep my desire for Alex in check, the preoccupation with him becomes stronger. It's like a fever: I hold imaginary conversations with him all the time. I've put up a mirror at home, to look at myself. Pulling up my T-shirt and admiring my concave stomach and pert rosy breasts, even I think I look beautiful, so why doesn't the bastard fancy me? I've just got

clear of the hang-ups I used to have about my appearance, and the eating disorders. Now I see them looming again. I'm humiliated by the fact that I haven't sensed an echoing response from him. If I knew Alex felt the same love and desire for me, it would help, I wouldn't feel so embarrassed and out of control.

I think I'm going to refer to him here as 'A' with a kiss next to it, for short. 'Ax'. I know he's a Taurean, because I guessed, then asked him. He did one of his abrupt switches from Caring to Sharply Contemptuous. I don't think it was just me trespassing over the line of his private domain: from something he muttered, he's hung-up about getting older. I don't care, I'd still have the hots for Ax if he was fifty.

****

Chloris

At the office, Chloris was reading an article in *The Psychotherapist* with interest.

'Sitting in the laundrette, I was obsessed with the idea that my clothes, painstakingly separated and put inside a clean machine drum (I had inspected it for several minutes, and sniffed it) were being washed in diarrohea. I stared through the transparent circular door at the pale clothing swinging round lazily clockwise then anticlockwise inside the washing machine. Better at least than the top loaders there used to be here in the mid-seventies. Then I thought that the laundry was not being washed at all, you weren't allowed to lift the iron lid to check.

I was always sniffing my hands and checking my shoes in case I had dog faeces on them. I once realised, really realised, how we are attached to the Earth, by logically thinking through how I was at risk of touching dog's muck on the pavement. Because I saw it, did not mean that I had bent down and touched it with my fingers, or transferred it to my face. In fact I was quite a long way away from it, even if standing over it, which I never did of course - I walked in a semi-circle around it. In this way I worked out that so long as

I walked upright, my feet were nearest to the dog's mess, my shins further away, my hands further away still. In fact, if I did not see it, perhaps I could stop thinking about it, as I did on a daily basis. I was not in danger of stepping in it accidentally, because I usually walked around staring at the ground. If I wanted to look up at the sky, or into the beautiful distance, or behind me, I stood stock still. It drove my friends mad, but here I was incapable of doing two physical things at once. The fact that I was performing myriad cerebral functions, working out my thoughts and desires and resisting compulsions, was naturally not apparent.

I had a horror generally of smelling unpleasant. Shit was uncontrollable. So was sick. Sometimes I wondered if I had been sick and hadn't noticed, that way madness lay. Bathing was a difficult process as there was a strict order of washing, bottom and genitalia first of course, then rinse hands and arms, lather them again, clean feet. In case one had Athlete's Foot, which could cause Non Specific Urethritis (this fear applied more in the days when I had a lot of different sexual partners), then one did the armpits after rinsing, with freshly lathered soap… and so on. At least it was easier now I had a shower at home. Previously, in myriad chilly rooms with tiny sinks and cold water it had been more difficult to wash properly. I had felt tired and resentful in my teens about the need for all this washing. I had had to do it furtively too, otherwise my mother stood outside the bathroom door and worried. Then I washed all over twice a day, at least now it's only once. Nowadays I'm so much better that I only wash my hair every two or three days.

The thoughts of those with OCD are horrendous. In the split second of passing a pushchair, you may wonder if you have intentionally impaled the infant's eye on the corner of your sharp tube ticket – just imagine passing thousands of people on your daily route to work, or just when out going to meet someone socially and experiencing a sharp anxiety and accompanying horrifying scenario for each one. I was constantly turning to stare at the back of un-wounded and generally oblivious strangers, their minds caught in their own concerns: Why didn't she ring me? How can I get him to pay

*me the money he owes me? Why doesn't the bastard contact
the girls? How come she got promoted?*

To die by one's own hand better. That thought helped me a
lot in childhood, when I had different but even more
excoriating anxieties – I often broke into cold sweats and felt
nauseous dread. I was startlingly pale and when people
remarked upon it, my mother decreed that I have a daily
spoonful of Malt Extract. To the outside in, when what was
desperately needed was for the inside to come out into the
healthy sunlight. Perhaps she thought that the Malt Extract
would gum up my mouth and voice so that the thoughts would
safely be sealed in.

I surveyed the endless years ahead of me and worried that I
would kill people, or already had murdered some - the thought
of suicide was my solace. I was obsessed with death and
murder and believed myself evil, as that was safest, any
thoughts to the contrary were quickly rejected. I was
convinced that other people would not like me if they knew
what I was really like. Everyone would turn against me, and
I'd deserve it as everything was my fault.

Until my mid-thirties I was prone to interrogating people when
anxious, often about something that sounded trivial, but which
had a huge bearing on my inner, concealed, anxiety about
something totally different. People were thus surprised (I
usually concealed all fear and anxiety beneath flippancy)
frightened, annoyed, estranged or worried by this abrupt
change in behaviour and the different side of my personality it
revealed. It felt impossible to tell them the big worry of the
moment. I felt that if I did that I would scream the world down
with distress, as well as thinking that they were judging my
ever after, so that every time they spoke I would assume they
were referring to my huge anxiety of that time, and I would go
into the cycle of dread and despair again. I realised much
later that the interrogations I subjected people to when I was
panic-stricken, were a vain quest for reassurance. I guess
that it was partly due to never being allowed to express
anxiety, or to talk about my problems during my childhood. I'm
pretty sure in retrospect that my mother had OCD: some
therapists suggest that there is evidence of several different

reasons for OCD, including genetic causes and learned behaviour.

I didn't realise I had OCD until I heard someone speaking on a television programme last year, and experienced Epiphany. For the first time it felt as though someone was speaking directly to me. As a lot of my life has been spent concealing my condition, I was obviously blocking any such realisation before. My parents couldn't, or wouldn't, ever discuss my anxieties.

Due to low self-esteem, and everything poisoned by my belief of being undeserving, I have lived in much sub-standard accommodation. Because I believed I did not have the right to judge, I often used to associate socially with people whose behaviour and views I sometimes had difficulty coping with.

At least I can touch people now in a normal manner. But if I suddenly feel panic I don't touch them at all, it's not worth the ensuing anxiety. From 14 or 15 I was scared to touch people, even boyfriends, in case I harmed them. From an early age, I was paranoid about anyone I knew to have health problems and very anxious if physically near them. I would feel very tempted to do something that would harm them, then worried frantically in case I had done it. This cut out future professions such as being a doctor or nurse, in case I gave someone the wrong medicine 'deliberately'.

I never felt overtly angry as a teenager and I wondered why not. Most people seemed to have vitriolic opinions about other people and situations. I found it very difficult to be judgmental about others when I believed I was so bad. In retrospect I think my anger was tamped down and denied, too 'dangerous' to express, along with the violent or bizarre thoughts I tried desperately not to think. Obviously all this made it very difficult for me to communicate in any real sense, apart from sociable, flippant, drunken interaction with other people. I also occasionally became violent when drunk. A sign of healthiness nowadays is that I may well exclaim 'I'll kill so-and-so!' in anger or amusement, without any anxiety, or thought of actually doing so.

Of course, to an onlooker the rituals of OCD can appear comical. To the sufferer, it is utterly hellish to be mocked or laughed at. One already feels incredibly conspicuous, whether this is the case or not. Imagine discovering your own worst fear has come true, then apply this feeling to every onslaught of OCD panic.

I found cognitive behavioural therapy a very different process to the type of general therapy I had participated in, on a one-to-one basis with three different therapists, for several years previously. The CB therapist had heard similar thoughts and anxieties to mine before. This is something that I find astonishing about OCD, that it is manifested in similar thoughts by very different individuals. Early on, the therapist briskly informed me that if I had 'contamination' fears he personally could not work with that. It would probably mean 'a nice spell in hospital'. Fortunately I could disabuse him of this notion: I've heard both positive and negative things about being treated in hospital for OCD.

I located my therapist through BACUP, I would not use anyone not medically accredited. By definition it is a frightening and sensitive process, letting some stranger inside one's thoughts. I was disgusted by the exorbitant fees charged by some of the practitioners on the list. It is immoral to charge more for working with a patient with mental illness than one suffering from a physical disability. I had doubts about working with a male therapist, as I thought the sexual/gender equation might complicate the process. In the event, he might as well have been a door wedge – as soon as one is working through painful procedures, the small issue of gender ceases to matter much. In fact, it was useful in enabling me to work through some difficulties I had had previously interacting with men. (And he did enable doors to be opened and remain so.)

I imagine it is akin to 'coming out' for a gay person, there is still a stigma in our society attached to being labelled mentally ill. Maybe because it is linked to lack of control, whereas I am the most controlling person I know - 'bossy' is too kind. I've happily 'come out' to old friends, who look at me with incomprehension or sympathy.

As an academic in my forties, I am appalled that firstly, that I did not realise much sooner what I was suffering from. Secondly, about the lack of public awareness, also publicity, concerning a condition that apparently affects one in six people (including children) to a lesser extent and one in 50 to a disabling degree. I have to add that I don't know if these statistics are true, as I have a lot of research to do on my condition now. Not much seems to have been performed thus far by the medical establishment and that which has, has mainly occurred in the years since the late '60s.

It's a double-edged sword, realising and accepting that you have a mental illness, but I am deeply relieved to have emerged from decades of terrible feelings of isolation. One of the most strange and moving experiences of my life was to attend an annual OCD Conference at Imperial College, London and realise that I was in a full Lecture Theatre with many hundreds of fellow sufferers. They all appeared totally sane.

Chloris slowly closed the journal and laid it in her 'Out' tray. Undine? Pondering, she went to the coffee machine.

****

Bubbles

Sitting on the floor of her room, Bubbles opened a new exercise book. She fantasised about Ax reading the romance she was writing, recognising her feelings for him and then acting on them.

Anthony showed no desire to leave. He drank his coffee with every sign of appreciation, lazing in an armchair, long legs stretched out. His dark gleaming shoes were of hand-stitched leather; they probably cost the same as she was paid for a fortnight's work, thought Ursula. Anthony looked curiously at her drawings and oil paintings hanging on the walls.
'Where did you buy these?' he asked, moving easily across the sitting room to look more closely. 'They're very good.'

'I did them,' Ursula admitted reluctantly. She wanted to add, but I don't any longer because Geoff sneered at them. Geoff was a proper artist. Ursula had gone out with him for three years, artistic temperament and all, until just eight months ago when she had chanced upon him in a passionate embrace with Jane, her best friend. Soon afterwards she discovered that Geoff had been secretly seeing Jane for more than a year.

Anthony saw Ursula's eyes fill with tears. 'I think you'd better go,' she said huskily. She hurried across the room blindly towards the hall and front door. She heard Anthony put his cup down abruptly, then he was beside her, filling the hall with his presence. He was so close she could smell his discreet aftershave.
'Goodness' he said gently. Ursula felt him lifting her chin with his finger until she was forced to look into his blue eyes. No longer cold, they looked down at her in smiling sympathy.
'Can I help?'
'It's okay. Really.' said Ursula blinking hard. She suddenly realised his hands were holding her shoulders. His light touch was sending treacherous waves of pleasure through her body, her knees felt weak.
Her hair, now dry, slid forward in a scented shining curtain over his fingers. All was silent, only they existed. His eyes were dark and unfathomable as he looked down at her. Ursula swayed towards him, closing her eyes; Anthony looked down at her. Suddenly he stepped back so abruptly that she almost fell. Ursula's eyes flicked open in shock, she stared at him.
'I must go' Anthony said huskily, his face set in harsh lines. Disbelievingly Ursula heard the front door click shut, and his footsteps retreating. Dazed, she returned to the sitting room and burst into tears. Anthony had seen her practically fainting into his arms - and been horrified. Well, now she had to move out, and quickly. But where?

To Ursula's surprise she slept well, but waking she winced as she remembered the events of the evening before. The question of where to move to loomed large once more. Although very dutiful, she did not feel relaxed with her parents; requesting to stay with them was not an option. She often felt that she looked after them, rather than the other way round. She didn't feel able to turn to her selfish younger sister, Elaine, either. Elaine lived miles away in Newcastle, and was madly in love with her new husband.

When the 'phone rang, it was a welcome distraction from her thoughts. It was her friend, Fatima. Fatima's voice rang exuberantly in Ursula's ear:

'Hi Ursula, how's it going?'

'Hello Fatima.'

'Hey what's up? You don't sound your usual happy self,' Fatima said with concern.

Ursula related the saga of losing her job as lightly as she could, interrupted by exclamations from her friend about the awfulness of men - particularly one called Anthony. 'I don't have enough savings to learn computing packages to try and get work Temping.' Ursula explained. She didn't say anything about financially helping her parents. 'Anyway I like my work, I don't think I'd like sitting in an office'.

'I'm sure something will come up soon,' Fatima soothed.

'Have you heard of any flats to rent? I don't want to stay here - Anthony's my landlord.'

'No... Unless of course... There is the arrangement I'm always nagging you about?' said Fatima teasingly.

'No no, I couldn't' said Ursula for the umpteenth time, since her friend had first raised the idea three months earlier.

'Oh well, never mind. I was just ringing to ask if you want to come to Whiteleys, to the cinema with us this afternoon. You know you like Ali, and he's potty about you.'

That's what I'm worried about, thought Ursula. 'He is a really nice person' she said weakly.

'I know, but you can't face a marriage of convenience to him. Oh Ursula, it would only mean living with him for a year so he could stay in the country.' pleaded Fatima. 'And it would solve both yours and Ali's problems: you could stay at his Knightsbridge flat, it's lovely there. Then you divorce or annul it or whatever. What more could you want?'

Ursula sighed; this was the most pressure Fatima had put on her yet. Ali was a distant relative of Fatima's; he was handsome, cheerfully irresponsible, loved having fun - she almost wished she could feel more for him than amused affection. Ursula knew Fatima was partly matchmaking, hoping a marriage of convenience would soften into love between them. But Geoff had left Ursula untrusting and disillusioned. Romantic love, pah! Suddenly Ursula caught herself up short and laughed. At this rate she'd be a lemon-sucking man-hater by the time she was twenty-five.

Ali's brown eyes lit up as she hurried up to him and Fatima outside the cinema;
'Hello gorgeous Ursula - will you marry me?' He kissed her hand with a flourish. As usual, he was wearing expensive casual clothes; Ursula had to admit he was handsome. Why couldn't she feel love or even attraction for Ali, who seemed so keen on her? He was now looking rather too appreciatively at her trim figure and glossy hair.
'Ali, don't be silly' she laughed. 'I live in hope' he said only semi-jokingly. As they sat in the darkness watching a Hollywood rom-com, Ursula was tempted for the first time to accept. She fought her uneasiness: so long as she was very clear from the outset that they were only platonic friends, it could work out well. It wasn't necessarily ethical, but it wasn't hurting anyone. It would help Ali and please Fatima. Her self-imposed payments to her parents loomed large in her mind - it would be heaven not to have to worry about letting them down, or about where to live. It was not as though she wanted to marry anyone else, after all. She hadn't even been out with anyone since Geoff. Ursula relaxed slightly, and began to watch the film.

As they all drank Cappucinos at a small Italian cafe afterwards, Ursula took a deep breath. It was now or never: 'Okay Fatima, Ali,' she said quietly in a voice she didn't recognise 'I'll do it.'
'Oh that's brilliant!' exclaimed Fatima, then remembering where they were, paid the bill and hustled them out into the street. Ali's face was alight with smiles: 'Let's all go back to my place and discuss it' he said, hailing a black cab.

Back at Ali's mansion flat, Ursula felt as though she was acting in a play. Fatima and Ali were busily discussing arrangements. Now the decision was made, Ursula felt very peculiar rather than relieved.

'Ursula, I'll type out all the details of yours and Ali's lives for you both to learn, ready for the authorities, so that they'll believe you are really in love.'
Ursula gave herself a mental shake: someone other than her seemed to be trying to listen to Fatima and to take things in. Fatima realising Ursula was in a state of shock, laughingly encouraged her to explore the flat. After all it was to be her home for the next twelve months. Ursula wandered around the sumptuous two-floored flat, trying not to be overwhelmed by the grandeur of high ceilings edged with ornate cornices, the heavy swagged curtains shading enormous bay windows, expensive wallpaper and Victorian furniture. The pristine white kitchen was an interior designer's dream, but the entire flat felt like a stage set, she thought, it was too perfect. The sound of the traffic outside was a subdued hum; Ursula's feet sank silently into the blue carpet.

****

Bubbles

Clocks at home were always ten minutes slow – should have been a century slow. Nothing modern entered the house until after I'd left, lugging my bin bags along the village lanes in the early morning to the railway station, and thence to Oxford. I'd told Grania I was moving out the night before as she lay in the other single bed a couple of feet away in the darkness. Somehow I didn't manage to tell her before, there was so little real communication.

In the event I was to move my belongings into a small bedsit in Oxford, surviving living within in four walls for three years. Thence to London, to the large luxurious home of professionals in Islington, known to one of the families I cleaned for, to a bare small bedroom. Finn drove me and my bin-bags there in a van, then whizzed off to meet with friends elsewhere in London. I didn't see him again for several months. As the balding conventional husband carried one of my boxes of clothes (a bag had split) up the stairs, he suddenly realised that his large nose was nestling in my black suspender belt lying on top. He blushed crimson as he hurriedly lifted his head and placed the box on a chest of drawers. A hook on the suspender belt caught on his collar. Panicking, he fought with it and detached himself with a tearing sound. 'Oliver, Oliver!' could be heard, floating melodically and crossly up the stairs. As he hurried down to his haggard wife - she was a doctor - I sat on the bed and stared at the blank white painted wall and felt unutterably lonely.

After that I moved excitedly to a cheap room in a terraced house in East London inhabited by two sensible students and a peculiar be-spectacled guy called Kevin. The latter used to chuck his chip fat into the bramble-filled tiny back garden. An alternative version of 'Lord of the Flies' could have been filmed there. Of all the small front gardens in the street, only one had any flowers: a single red luxuriant rose. It glowed like a drop of blood amongst all the grey concrete and grime. Our garden had the only tree: dogs used to visit from miles around. The house was on the 73 bus route to my English Literature university course, which I didn't buckle down to, thinking how great it was to have a loan. Of course analysis has its place, but I didn't agree with picking apart literature that other people had already done to extinction, once I'd realised that's all it was. Trying to find things in the text that the author had never meant and would be surprised to learn, just to give other people something to do with their lives, rather than create something themselves. I spent my loan recklessly on clothes and socialising then, bored, went to work at a fashionable nightclub, rubbing shoulders with the famous.

I became a North London Nomad, I went on to live in eleven different places in seven years. I loved London, a place of dreams and infinite possibilities, but I was on the run from myself, or my difficulty with asserting myself with housemates, or I'd move somewhere bargain cheap. Occasionally I moved from boredom, to distract myself, to use up my bursts of manic energy, to fill in the empty swathes of time that other people had filled for them by family relationships. I enjoyed scrubbing out and painting some dingy hell-hole, hanging my paintings carefully on new walls, transforming the space into an airy light haven and a home for a successor. I had a hell of a lot of baggage too (in every sense) so would drag bin bags and my aquarium around on public transport when I wasn't offered lifts by acquaintances. I wanted to appear totally independent of my family, so that they couldn't say that I'd failed in any way - not that they offered any help. And oddly, I've ended up at Einstein Road. In fact, come to think of it, I've been here a year and a half, a long time for me, though I still wouldn't call it home. But trust me to do the opposite of the seven-year-itch.

The trouble with standing still for once, not running from myself and my thoughts, is that a tsunami of anxiety, guilt and remorse is relentlessly gathering in a mountainous wave on the horizon, moving in fast towards me standing like a statue on the shingle.

****

Einstein Road

There was a Co-op Housing meeting in session at Einstein Road when Bubbles entered the crowded sitting-room with Marius, she'd forgotten all about it. She and Marius had been at his house, in his room high under the eaves. Brought abruptly back to earth, Bubbles now hesitated shyly in the doorway of the room. There were people perched all over the furniture and sitting on the floor. Alistair the Arrogant, an ex-public school boy with cultivated Estuary accent, was sitting upright on the sofa, pontificating. He seemed to be talking about work that needed doing at Rugby Street, and how Art hadn't contacted the Council about a grant when he'd said he would, so now they'd probably lost the chance to apply. Art retorted that he'd understood that Alistair had had it all under control, at the last meeting. Alistair demanded to know where the Minutes were for the last meeting, everyone looked at Bubbles. Sorry, she mumbled, I forgot. Do you need me to take notes now? Has anyone got a pencil...?
'Rosalie's doing them,' said Nick curtly, smiling across at Rosalie. Rosalie looked complacently down at her shorthand pad. Her black biro sped neatly across the page. Bubbles saw a small empty space on the floor and apologetically made for it, smiling vaguely, stepping over legs and prickling with self-consciousness. When she eventually plucked up

courage to look around, Marius had vanished. She noticed that Helena, Chloris, Matilda, Rosalie, Alistair's girlfriend Sophie, Vivienne, Nick, Finn, India and Art were present. They were discussing the Treasurer's Report. Sophie announced the amounts currently in the Bank accounts, then began reading out a list of members who owed rent arrears. Bubbles was surprised to learn that she owed £420, more even than Finn.

'There needs to be a limit on rent arrears,' Vivienne was saying.

'How would you implement it?'

'That if it reaches, say £500, people have to move out, otherwise they're just taking the piss.'

There was an outcry. 'Why not become a Fascist and have done with it!' someone could be heard saying amongst the protests.

'It doesn't affect you if I owe money,' Finn said calmly, 'Actually, the trouble is, it does,' retorted Alistair, glancing slyly at Vivienne, whom he fantasised about on her motorbike. 'When we apply for grants and stuff, they usually ask to see the books, to see that members are behaving responsibly and that we have some income. For fuck's sake Finn, your rent's only 30 quid a week!'

There was an uncomfortable silence as everyone, including Alistair, realised he'd gone too far. Finn looked at him contemptuously.

Bubbles realised her stomach muscles were clenched hard with anxiety.

'I've got another job,' she said nervously, 'I could pay instalments ...'

There was an unconvinced silence and she realised that people were avoiding looking at her.

'You said you'd do that, oh, this time last year,' said Alistair. Chloris, who disliked Alistair intensely, suddenly said: 'I can lend you the money Undine, we'll talk about it later.'

Bubbles couldn't believe her ears; she stared across the room at Chloris, who looked embarrassed. Alistair looked disappointed, then meaningfully across at Vivienne. Bubbles saw Vivienne shrug slightly in response.

'Right well, um, what's next on the Agenda? Oh yeah, the wall at Bell Street-'

****

Gabriel

It's my lunch-hour; I'm eating my sandwiches and fruit bought from the hospital shop outside in the front courtyard, adjacent to a busy road, catching some free Spring sunshine and carbon monoxide. I'm sharing the space with patients wearing dressing-gowns attached to mobile drips and having a fag, doctors and nurses in uniform also smoking, porters eating apples and relatives sitting chatting.
'Oi!' bellows a girl aged about eleven, strolling along with her friend, both kitted out expensively in the latest logos.
'Don't say "Oi!" Tara, it's rude. "Say "Excuse me mister", if you want to get my attention," retorts a dark-haired man. The girls laugh, unabashed.

I'm trying to think of money-making ventures, so I'm writing down some of my invention ideas:

- Energy-generating road' on cantilevers which energises vehicles, cutting down on pollution

- All in one hand-powered-by-trigger remote for DvD, TV, radio, blinds, etc.

- Self-cleaning bath – flushes like loo

- Catflaps with different frames of curtains, e.g Victorian flounces etc.
NOTE: Torquil is keen on this idea. In fact he's been talking to Helmut about it, who runs a trendy gift shop. You know the sort of thing, witty mirrors, Alessi anything, and silver corkscrews.

Other ideas include:

- Cat and dog flaps that clean the animals, with brushes at the sides and a moving walkway to get the mud off their paws.
- Cycling codpieces/aerodynamic helmet - ho ho.

- Floating bed - user wears suit of repelling magnets above magnetic mattress.

NOTE: Research potential difficulty of getting out of bed without painfully falling on to floor.

- Sewage line instead of plimpsoll line, indicating when boat tank requires emptying. In fact having a transparent tank might be good? Perhaps not.

- Contraption that could be bolted onto boats without engines, so as to attach temporary outboard motors.

NOTE: It would be worth making one of those just to see Torquil's expression, as he arrived home in the early hours to an empty mooring.

My jottings are abruptly interrupted by seeing the husband of an Indian woman whom I interviewed this morning, prior to her MRI scan. I shrink down on my bench, slide my sunglasses on and practice auditioning as The Invisible Man. It transpired the patient had an IUD she hadn't told her husband about. Florence, who fortunately speaks Urdu, broke it up. They're walking past me now, her a couple of paces behind him, both of them stony-faced.

As you've guessed, I'm working in the Scanning Unit, apparently the mention of guns was a joke, Rob Roy being such a wit. Florence, with whom I work, is a darling. She's been here for eleven years and loathes Lasain, her Manager. She adores her boss's boss though, who also views the reviled Lasain with contempt, so that's all right. Florence recognised me from the sitcom immediately, and is thrilled in an undemonstrative way. She keeps helping me, which makes me feel guilty and inadequate when she's so busy herself, plus she's already fed-up with having helped a succession of Temps who've left (the wages for the permanent job are pitiful) or been sacked. Lasain only dismisses the efficient ones, to Florence's fury, because they make her look inefficient, so I'm safe. The doctors gabble on the audio tapes, which makes the medical terminology impossible to hear, let alone spell. I became worried because I lost some of the medical reports on tape. I wish I didn't understand the wider ramifications of my tiny, frantic part in the huge machine that is … The Hospital! Cue for creepy music and 'Rocky Horror Show' storm.

Luckily the MRI Unit is situated near the entrance, otherwise I'd be permanently lost, instead of merely when I have to go to the Admin. Office on Fridays to hand in a copy of my timesheet. It's on the second floor, but can only be accessed by a particular staircase. I realised this last week after I'd wandered around the third floor for 45 minutes between locked sections. I met the same builder up a ladder twice, he'd spilt paint on the floor which made it very slippery, good job he's working in a hospital. I'd asked someone to hold the swing door and it locked behind me, and I don't have any of the security swipe cards.   Florence kindly came to find me before I starved to death, for which I am undyingly grateful.

One of my tasks is to interview patients, to discover whether they have anything metal on or inside them. If this isn't removed it grows hot and moves when the patient is inside the huge scanning machine. Neither the patients – who are almost universally pleasant people, why doesn't Fate dish out cancer scares to more bastards for a change? – nor I, understand half the questions on the form. I can't even pronounce some of the words. At least someone has thoughtfully put the number of the Crash Team on the Scanning Room door underneath the 'Danger!' and 'Radioactive' signs, so that if I do accidentally send someone in with a Pacemaker they'll stand some chance of being saved.

Torquil rang me at work today; I wasn't thrilled as I'd given him the number for emergency use and he sounded as though he'd rung for a chat.
'I've ripped out all that nasty old damp wood in the kitchen and that ghastly cupboard under the sink.'
'Oh.' My heart sank.
'We thought you'd be pleased Gabriel!' He sounded sulky.
'We?'
'Robin and I worked terribly hard, and we've having to rub in gallons of hand cream now, even though we wore Marigolds.'
'Marigold's what?' Torquil used to know a Drag Queen by that name; she certainly wore a lot of rubber.

'Ha, ha.'

'Um, thanks … So what's the sink standing on?'

'You should have seen what was at the back of the cupboard under the work surface, the smell-'

'Torq,'

''Sorry, line's breaking up,'

'Torquil!'

'I beg your pardon?'

'Is.there.still a..sink. in. the. kitchen?'

'No, but there's the little one in the bathroom still of course, Rob rang Rory who's a really nice plumber and he's promised to come round as soon as his present job finishes-' He ran out of breath.

I'd misjudged Torquil, it was an emergency. I rested my head on the desk.

'Robin says I can stay at his house until the work's done. Are you still there? Oh, by the way, the gas bottle has run out for the cooker, I've arranged for Roores to deliver a new one.'

'Oh, thanks.'

'Yes, they can do it early on Friday morning.' Today is Monday.

Soon after the call, I had to dash across the reception area to answer the 'phone on Florence's desk and took the audio machine crashing with me, I forgot the earplugs were in my ears. At least it made Maisie the radiologist laugh.

****

Therapy Session

'We're going somewhere else today Undine.' Ax was standing in the centre of the lamp-lit basement room.

'Hold on a sec.' He looked round the comforting room, crouched to rifle through cardboard files stacked against the wall with initials on them.

'Here we are.' He lifted my file and I self-consciously preceded him up the steps to the pavement. 'Just across here, I don't like spending the whole of my time in a basement. Anyway, as you saw, my research is spread out across the floor in there.'

He was running up a wide flight of steps to an imposing front door, heavy with stained glass. He held the door open and I entered a grand echoing hall; I heard him lock the front door behind us.

'Why did you do that?' I asked timidly.

'I like to be sure my clients won't run away.' He grinned disarmingly. Ax moved ahead and through a doorway on the left. 'You sit here,' he was indicating a chair that faced away from the main part of a huge sitting room. 'So that you don't get distracted by all the things in here.'

Once we began the session I wasn't distracted by Ax's appearance, which is all that will affect me. He is not to know, but I'm used to expensive houses and *objets d'art* after going out with Simon.

'I'm scared, coming here.'

'Why, because it's a new place?'

'Partly, I preferred the basement because it felt cosy.'

'Are you frightened of anything else?'

'Fear of the unknown,' I muttered. I said bravely: 'I don't understand how the therapy will progress and you won't tell me.'

Ax was silent.

'I feel that it's going too fast. I don't think you'll let me work the way I want to, is it possible so that I feel more in control? Why won't you just tell me the structure so that I know roughly what to expect week to week?'

'I do sometimes tell people the structure of the way in which we'll work. Lots of people with OCD want to know.'

Well, wouldn't you? You wouldn't like to be out of control. I didn't say this, although the thought was so loud I wondered he couldn't hear it.

'I'm not telling you, because I think it might adversely affect the way in which we work together.' I suddenly wondered if he wasn't telling me because he hasn't done the work and formulated a structure. The thought was gone before I could deal with it.

'It slows us down if I'm really scared.'

After a pause he said: 'You can lead the sessions, Undine.' I don't believe him, we'll see.

'I said last time you could work the way you want to and I'd be quiet. But I'm not, am I?'

He looked wryly at me.

'This chair is so uncomfortable,' I said at one point. I couldn't sit upright without balancing on the front of the seat, as the Indian chair back sloped backwards. It felt uncomfortable, and I felt vulnerable having to lean back so far. Apparently there are chairs made for men and, differently, for women. It's to do with thigh length whether you're comfortable, I bet it was a man's seat. Feels like a man's room, everything grandiose and displayed to impress.

'Let's change then,' Ax offered with alacrity, springing up from his usual place, a velvet *chaise longue*.

'A reversal of roles,' I said lightly, after seating myself rather shyly on it. It wasn't much better and my legs aren't short. Is there a female equivalent of Freud? I bet there isn't, because furniture hasn't been created for her.

Suddenly Ax asked: 'Undine, why would I not ring you back?' I rang him twice before the session – a major feat, astonishing what obsessive love can do - and left messages. 'Because you hate my guts' I said jokingly. His face changed with shock and he struggled not to laugh. I love shattering that impassivity. 'Try again,' he said gently.

'That was a joke,' I said pleadingly, but could see that Ax didn't dare believe me

'I rang because if it had been a good-bye session, I couldn't have come today. I would have found it too difficult to enter the house in case I touched something in a way I wasn't happy with. It would worry me intolerably afterwards.'

'Undine, why ever did you think it would be good-bye session?' He was half-laughing.

'Because we didn't resolve the situation last time.'

He stopped laughing. 'I would always tell you if it was going to be the last session.'

'How it actually hit me, was that I was worried in case I had touched the underneath of this seat and left a message there.' I babbled, sweating with embarrassment and anxiety.

He looked strangely relieved. 'What would make you happy about that now?'

'If I could touch it again.'

So, eventually, I reach down and touched the chair, for a split second, and we discussed my anxiety ratings and my thoughts while I was doing it.

It's a drawback that Ax never feels he can joke with me, I'm so much better than I used to be, that I can cope with coming to see him. As I was leaving, I said, 'I'm not as confident as I appear.'
'You don't say,' Ax drawled, which made my face relax into a natural smile for what felt like the first time.

Why am I so obsessed by him? Perhaps I'm going mad. Perhaps I've transferred too great burden of worry and anxiety onto Ax and so think about him too much now. I suppose it has to be less distressing than worrying about my problems, but it feels weird. Christ took up humans' burdens ... I hold conversations with Ax in my head all the time now, it's as though he's in there with me. I was wearing a long skirt last session, split so that it showed off my newly sun-tanned legs. Ax didn't look once. He doesn't care about my appearance, it's my mind he's interested in. I don't think he'll be able to cope. Fasten your new-seat belt, Sunshine, you're in for a bumpy ride.

I couldn't face asking for an extra ten minutes to be added on to the session, to make up for last week.

****

Alexander

I'd better check the rest of Undine's manuscript for references to me, then I can get shot of it.

ARIES

Oh I remember, pornographic astrology.

Aidan whimpered in ecstasy, a wolf in accountancy clothing. Soon afterwards, they surfed orgasm simultaneously (Matilda operatically) and collapsed on to the rug. Aidan had appeared at Einstein Road six weeks before to audit the accounts. He was conspicuous by his difference to most males who appeared at Einstein Road, armoured as he was by a conservative suit, steady income, professional reticence and bearing a slim black briefcase. Matilda found him exotically attractive and asked him if he could repair her DvD player. She wondered what would happen as they climbed the stairs to her bedroom on the third floor. Aidan carefully rolled up his white shirt sleeves, exposing long fair hairs on his arms. He gave his opinion regarding the machine, but failed to repair it, whilst Matilda wearing a mini dress lounged against the wardrobe staring at him admiringly.

The woman's insatiable.

Seemingly indifferent to these signals, Aidan returned downstairs; polished, black, leather shoes echoing against the bare boards. He spread out the Bank statements and a few other dog-eared documents that had been unearthed regarding the Co-op accounts, on the circular kitchen table.

Matilda, intrigued, retired to have a bath. She lay idly in the warm water in the gloom, observing the water distortion that rendered her toes stubby or elongated as she swayed amongst the ripples. There was a click in the passage. Suddenly apprehensive, she sat up. Glancing at the locked door, she thought she saw a white flicker through the frosted glass panels. Matilda reached for the towel lying on the floor. Rising with a rush of water, she hurriedly wrapped it around her.

While Matilda was recalling this, the vengeful courier behind Rosalie's car was knocked flying by a red C10 bus swinging round into John Islip Street. Seeing his body part company from the bike and skid across the pavement, Rosalie smiled triumphantly in the car mirror. Matilda emerging from her fantasy, saw the front gardens of an imposing white Regency terrace spasmodically revealed through gaps in Box hedging.

That's where Rupert lives. I used to think my brother in law didn't like me, but he's been won over

One day she would live somewhere like that, decided Matilda.

Hardly likely!

She'd ditch Dion and-

Rosalie was speaking.

'Sorry Rosie, I missed that.'

'I'm so glad I've split. I want to enjoy myself and maybe find someone new – before my boobs become like empty sacks drying over a wall.'

Matilda laughed, thinking they looked like heat-seeking missiles pointing straight ahead.

Vic and Vince were in total agreement, crammed side by side on a plush seat on a No.11 double-decker bus.

'Get a load of that.'

They stared down appreciatively at Rosalie's cleavage as it drew alongside, then accelerated away. As the window steamed up, Vince wiped it with a large red palm breathing loudly through clogged nostrils. Alrick, seated behind them, was feeling hung-over and bus-sick. His condition was exacerbated by Vic and Vince's unique aura of chip fat, nicotine and stale sweat.

'D'you know life?'

'Na. What's it like?

Alrick decided to miss an interesting philosophical discussion and walk the last mile.

'It's good.'

'Yeah?'

Alrick rose with difficulty, clutching at the pole. His face was pale and clammy.

'It's a new Club. Over New Cross way.'

He giddily swayed past them towards the door.

'Get a load of 'im,' Vince said disapprovingly as the bus screeched to a halt.

Vic grunted in agreement and shifted carefully inside his black leather jacket. As they pulled away from the kerb Alrick could be seen toppling into a sooty hedge.

'I was down the dog track last night, back on firm now.'

'How much d'you win?'

'Monkey.'

'Nice one. Coming back to my gaff?'

'Na, taking young Sharon over McDumps for Bulls-Eyes-in-Batter.'

Ugh.

Matilda's relationship with Alrick was quite different to the one she had with Dion: more like falling in love with the boy next door. He was wholesome, smelt sweet including when he smelt of dope, wore her cast-off jumpers and jeans and bathed daily in soap-free water. Despite his ablutions, Alrick was usually covered in a fine layer of sawdust as he made musical instruments. He used silence as a social weapon at parties and shared a large Victorian house in a quiet street on the other side of Kentish Town. Alrick existed on a cheap, wholesome, diet of vegetables and bread, his red-knuckled large hands dreamily scraping the dirt off potatoes in a white enamel basin of water in the kitchen sink. His thick brown shoes looked too big for him, he was short and muscular with creamy skin, red hair and eyes like pale blue china. Usually they made love in his single bed in his brightly painted room under the eaves, amongst the tops of soughing trees. Matilda liked sitting on the floor of his bare room looking at the murals flowing round the walls and listening to the wood pigeons cooing above them in the loft. 'Are you thinking about sex again?' Rosalie's tone was harsh. 'Yep,' said Matilda happily.

Towering vertically, the former British Gas headquarters on Millbank had been re-clad in greenish glass and transformed with the extravagant use of soft furnishings and Smeg kitchen appliances into palatial apartments. Aidan, housed in a penthouse on the seventeenth floor, was also thinking about sex with Matilda. The flat was an investment of his father's, and unbeknownst to him and his son, formerly the office canteen. Aidan had enjoyed dallying with Matilda, but thought he really preferred men, despite stubble rash. Holding a post-coital brandy he idly stroked a sleeping Murdoch's leg and surveyed wondrous views of the London skyline and Thames barges sliding along the brown gelatinous river below. He admired Rosalie's car from his lofty viewpoint, whilst wondering about the faint odour of boiled cabbage that permeated his new flat.

It would be nice to read something pleasant.

Noisy torrents of vehicles surged alongside the sports car containing Matilda and Rosalie. Small groups of tourists dawdled along the wide, flagged pavement. Rosalie saw several young boys, in a cluster on the pavement. Two of them were pressing hard against the window of a small, empty, workman's café with their hands. They were pale and excited. A man walked past the group; another boy in a grubby anorak carrying a long pointed wooden stick broke away from the group, he looked uncertainly around, grinning, and caught Rosalie's approving look. She nodded towards the retreating pedestrian - Matilda was preoccupied, steering round a cyclist. The boy stabbed the man hard in the back of his bulky coat. The man spun round angrily, the group stared back silent with anticipation. The boy pursued him for a few yards along the pavement with the stick clutched like an arrow, then changed his mind and threw it wide. The stake fell into the road in front of the car with a dry clatter.

Thank heaven William is down for Eton.

As they cruised slowly onward, helplessly caught in the stream of traffic, a metre from Rosalie's door a beggar lay on the icy pavement. He watched the boys indifferently, half wrapped in his grubby sleeping bag, one red swollen hand clutching a can of cider. He was reflected in glass entrance doors barring warm vacant offices.
'This country!'
'Poor sod.' Matilda agreed.
But Rosalie was indicating orange covers thrown over the traffic lights as they approached crossroads. A dozen lanes of vehicles, with buses towering like scarlet whales above smaller fry, surged in bad-tempered waves in front of Vauxhall Bridge.
'We go left Rosalie, we don't cross the river.'
She was surprised by Rosalie's exaggerated relief. Another Routemaster bus roared past, causing hanging baskets suspended from lampposts to sway. Looking right before they roared left on to Millbank, Matilda saw blue and yellow cranes in Grosvenor Road high in the sky like furled peacocks. As Rosalie reached across and turned on the headlights, Matilda saw the metal cranes swing from horizontal to vertical against the grey clouds, in a perfect chorus line.

Matilda parked deftly on a single yellow line next to Ponsonby Place. Hugging themselves against the chilly wind, she and Matilda hurried past The Morpeth Arms. The Youngs pub sign creaked in the wind, the castle separated from the ram above, on a red and white striped background.

I met Wendy there once ...

The Ministry of Defence building loomed futuristically across the river, a forbidding green and mustard fortress. Red buses wended their way beneath road bridges on the opposite bank. 'Look, up here, at this statue, he's one of my favourites.' **'Not bad.' Rosalie squinted up at the bronze dancer leaping gracefully above their heads, supported by unfurling ribbon: 'Do they look like that in your ballet class?'** 'On a good day.'

Matilda stopped curiously in front of a large ornate building with a diminutive stone coat of arms above a small door. Rosalie, seeing effortlessly past the blank stare of the security camera, wondered whether to tell Matilda what was inside, then decided against it. Matilda remarked: 'Makes you paranoid, wondering who's watching you.' 'Couple of geeks,' thought Rosalie, glancing up. Kevin, on the receiving end of her basilisk stare, felt his heart thud unpleasantly. As they crossed Atterbury Street, the cameras hurriedly swivelled away.

The Tate appeared, set graciously back from the pavement amongst green lawns, a silvery stone palace, with colonnades flanking wide steps leading up to the grand entrance. Black and orange coloured hangings denoted a new exhibition: *Hieronymus Bosch supported by SniffDeclineKillem*, near bronze life-sized statues flanking the entrance level. Rosalie looked approving. On the right a bronze man wearing a winged helmet and little else, brandished a severed head and a sword. 'Is that a Gorgon's head?' 'Oh, I hope not!' exclaimed Rosalie, remembering relatives. 'No look, it's Andromeda.'

The blue and cream Italian ice-cream van parked at the bottom of the steps was doing brisk business with tourists, despite the cold weather. Nearby, a tramp was trying to stretch out on a narrow sloping red plastic bench in a transparent bus shelter. He kept falling off.
'Good installation,' said Rosalie watching, prepared to be impressed by the Tate.
'That's life imitating art,' said Matilda crossly.

They stumbled through revolving doors onto the black and white mosaic floor of the vestibule and into echoes. They passed beneath arches into a circular brightly-lit space beneath a lofty glass rotunda. Matilda wandered ahead into peaceful stone gallery space, donated by Lord Duveen of Millbank MCMXXXVII, the record of his philanthropy set in stone for posterity. Well thanks anyway my Lord, from this prole, thought Matilda fervently, staring at the high windows admitting truthful light through walls above her. The air subtly echoed with voices as in a peaceful church. Rosalie loathed the architecture though, so they went downstairs - Rosalie hurrying past a stained glass window - to drink Cappuccinos and eat Mars bars in the basement café.

I'll pop round to the café soon for an Expresso - I hope the pretty Italian girl's working today.

To Matilda's relief, Rosalie approved of the metal torso of 'The Rock Drill'. Her appreciation was not shared by Ron, a museum attendant. He asked her to stop stroking the sculpture (which was also enjoying it) only to experience a burning sensation in his throat.
'You have all this stuff for the blind; she's allowed to touch things,' Rosalie had protested loudly. She waved her arm disparagingly at a woman wearing headphones and following a metal strip on the floor with a white cane. A couple nearby looked at Rosalie askance. The woman was now walking towards a bronze sculpture of a naked man with an explanatory Braille plaque beneath.
'That's experimental, French, and we can't extend it to everyone or the sculptures would be harmed. She has to wear a glove if it's marble, young woman-.' Ron suddenly stopped. He clutched his throat and his eyes bulged.

Ron regaled his mates that evening in The Morpeth Arms at such length about his run-in with Rosalie, that they kindly told him to shut it. As Vic said, 'As if a bird's eyes could glow red! What are you like? Your turn to get a round in.'

'Wow the medieval imagination was really something, ' Rosalie said with such relish standing in front of a Bosch painting, that several visitors smiled.
'I have to go to the loo, meet you back here?' Matilda walked away.
Rosalie peered closely at *The Garden of Earthly Delights*. She nodded to one of the devils in the painting. It grinned at her ferociously, then prodded a naked human viciously in the eye with a stake. The woman screamed appallingly.
'See ya around Meph,' Rosalie whispered. She glanced round, Alrick was standing slightly behind her, staring incredulously. He looked fearfully from her to the painting and back again. Rosalie smiled charmingly, then saw Matilda returning.
'Let's go look at the religious stuff while we're here,' she said hurrying towards Matilda, tucking an arm through hers and swinging her round before she saw Alrick.
'I didn't know you were religious, Rosie.'
'I'm not, I just love seeing pain.'
They emerged from rooms hung with crucified Christs and tortured martyrs. Matilda felt nauseous, and Rosalie reinvigorated with a sacrilegious delight.
'Rosalie, I'm losing it. I thought one of those martyrs in that picture writhed just now.'
Rosalie licked her lips slowly. 'Did you?'
'Would you mind if we went? I don't feel like seeing any more – I've got museum malaise,' Matilda forced a laugh.

They emerged from the bright warmth of the Tate into cold twilight. Streetlights twinkled across the river like crystals in the velvety dusk
'Drink in town?'
'Nice of them to lay on a Turner sunset.'
They admired it from the relative warmth of the car. 'So where now?' asked Matilda revving the engine. 'How about Covent Garden?'

'You know, I heard that there's a good pub in the Strand ..? I haven't been to an English pub yet, it'd be a gas.'

'How's things, still in love with Dion?' Rosalie asked as they sat in the Coal Hole nursing brandies.

Matilda's thoughts reverted to her recent one-night stands with Aidan and Alrick.

Well, there are others ...'

'That's my girl!'

'I met two guys recently, Alrick and Aidan, weird names...'

'What are they? Vikings?'

'Maybe. Great at pillaging,' said Matilda with relish.

Rosalie felt a stab of jealousy as she tuned in to Matilda's thoughts. They'd only been brief liaisons though, and she could ensure that it was not repeated - not with Matilda anyway.

Meanwhile Matilda was hoping it would be – a perfect zipless fuck, squared, without any of that messy romantic stuff. What Dion didn't know wouldn't hurt him. She clinked glasses and drank brandy with Rosalie.

'That first guy, Aidan was it? What a ram!'

'He looked like a sheep to start with. Almost had me fooled!'

'Seriously Mat, I'm surprised you have time for work; perhaps you should do this for a living.'

Matilda looked sharply at Rosalie. 'What?'

'Hey, only kidding.'

'Well,' said Matilda more calmly, 'I did know someone once, Delia, she did it at the top end of the market, she got over £1000 a time.'

'Actually I know someone here, friend of Greg's, who runs something along those lines. Very discreet, classy stuff.'

'It's really risky though, going to guy's hotel rooms. Delia did say though that they seemed more scared of her, than the other way round.'

'Well, let me know if you change your mind, it's good money,' murmered Rosalie. Matilda looked thoughtful, then laughed. 'I like a straightforward bit of perversion as much as the next woman.'

Hadn't realised Undine was so ... knowledgeable.

Rosalie smiled appreciatively. 'You can charge extra for that – what shall we call your future offshore company account?'
'Bottom's Up!'
They clashed glasses to the future venture. Fiery glints inside the oily brandy flashed sombrely
'I don't know why you keep him on,'
'Who, Dion? I sometimes wonder, old swillbelly that he is.'
'You don't even usually drink, life's too short.'
'He used to be great when I started stripping at The Windmill. He was bored to death even then, spotlighting dancer's bits, and it's a job most guys would kill for.'
'You know why I'm here, in London, Mat? I was looking at this book of poems -
Rosalie stood up suddenly on the rungs of her stool and dramatically tossed back her dark hair. Men seated nearby turned admiringly.

But at my back I always hear
Time's winged chariot hurrying near;
And yonder all before us lie
Deserts of vast eternity.

Rosalie sat down with a thump, to scattered applause. She flashed a complacent smile: 'Living life, that's what it's about!'
'Yes, that's why I do some of the things I do – might die tomorrow. Let's have another drink to celebrate Living,' said Matilda, laughing.
'Yeah, I'll get them, I'll drive back.'
Rosalie went to the bar and bought herself a Coke and Matilda a double brandy.
'Fancy spoiling a good brandy with coke.'
'What the hell,' said Rosalie who had no intention of being arrested. 'Wanna look at Greg?'
'Oh yes! That's a smart 'phone.'
'Yeah the radio's cool too.' Rosalie flashed an image onto the tiny screen.
A handsome athletic man flashed white teeth in a tinny laugh, eyes screwed up against the sun.
'Is he on the 'phone now, then?' asked Matilda puzzled.
'Oh no, that was him ages ago. It's a film.'
'Nice. Better not let Murdoch see it, he's a bit light-fingered.'

'He's really something though, I wouldn't mind him light-fingering me.'

'Rosalie! He's with Bubbles,' said Matilda laughing.

Rosalie shrugged, then laughed:

'Hey, just joking, but they're not living together.'

She got up and strolled across to a jukebox.

Leader of the Pack blared forth.

'Hey Mat, fancy going to see *Die Hard 24* now, or the new Van Damme film?'

Without Rosalie's eyes fixed on her, Matilda suddenly felt exhausted. She found herself yearning for Dion and his integrity. The warm red lights in the pub seemed stifling. She pushed her glass away and struggled unsteadily to her feet, clutching at the table.

'I have to get back,' she said.

'Sure.'

Rosalie looked absently at a television, high in a corner of the room, an advertisement for 'Victory V' cough sweets filled the screen with brown oblong shapes.

Matilda said: 'Do you have them in the US? We used to see how thin we could suck them, in the church choir when I was a kid.' Matilda suddenly saw a shadow of a face on the wall. The nose hooked over to almost meet the sharp chin, hair writhing from the head like a halo of snakes. 'Hey Rosalie, you've turned into a witch.' She laughed.

Rosalie turned sharply. The shadow vanished. 'Charming!'

'Oh, but there was- Sorry. It must have been a trick of the light. Are you all right?'

'Not really,'

Rosalie folded her arms across her lower abdomen and bent forward on the banquette, hissing.

****

Bubbles

Bubbles was trying to read a novel on the sofa in the cold sitting-room. She was warm now that she had donned coat, mittens and a hat. Despite herself, her mind obsessively retained the image of Rosalie and Murdoch below her in the hall. Perhaps Rosalie had had a car accident, that was why she and Matilda hadn't returned yet. Hurriedly Bubbles

visualised Matilda as unhurt; Rosalie though was lying on the
road, neck broken. As with Isadora Duncan, perhaps that
velvet scarf had caught on something and cut off her air
supply. Bubbles dealt guiltily on this vision: Rosalie's swollen
blackened face, eyes filled with blood, the ambulance lights
strobing the freezing night, people in fluorescent jackets
under the street lamps, the car crumpled like paper-
She quickly tapped her book three times to show that she
didn't mean it. She started nervously as the poster on the
chimney breast peeled off the wall and crashed onto the
hearth. Bubbles reached for the 'phone on the floor and rang
Murdoch's number. Vivienne answered.

'Hello Bubbles, no I haven't seen him since you last called. I'll
just check if he's in his room,' she said coolly. Vivienne was
another woman who made Bubbles feel inadequate. With
disappointment she heard her knocking loudly on Murdoch's
door in the distance, then footsteps returning to the 'phone.
'No Bubbles, he's not back yet.'
'Um, would you mind-'
The receiver was firmly replaced.

Later Matilda made up a bed for Rosalie on the floor of the
whitewashed empty room at the end of the downstairs
corridor, Rosalie watched. They could see their breath as
Matilda spread sheets and the duvet on top of the inflatable
mattress. The darkness outside pressed against the un-
curtained window.

'I'll just get you a heater and lamp, that'll make it cosier in
here,' said Matilda apologetically, in the doorway. 'At least
there's a rug.'
'A lamp would be good, don't worry about the heater. Thanks
again, Mattie.'
Rosalie was pale beneath her tan. After Matilda left to see
Dion, she stood rigidly in the centre of the room, haggard
under the harsh light, breathing quickly. 'Hell!' she whispered.
She opened her door to check the passage was empty, then
hurried to the lavatory. There wouldn't be any children for the
Co-op to reject.
Upstairs, Bubbles, tossing and turning in bed, suddenly
smiled and relaxed into a deep sleep.

....

The following evening, Rosalie was alone in the sitting-room at Einstein Road. She picked up the 'phone and rapidly checked the last number called. It was local; taking a risk she pressed the button.

'Hello,' said Murdoch irritably. He'd just read an intense and angry letter from Bubbles about their relationship, questioning whether it had a future.

Know how he feels, Wendy's getting boring. I suppose Undine's not a bad writer if you like this sort of thing.

'Hi,' said Rosalie meaningfully.

'Who's this?'

'Rosalie.' She opened her laptop computer.

'Hello there,' he said intrigued. 'How did you get this number?'

'Oh, I have my ways,' she said flirtatiously, pressing keys. A picture of a necklace filled the screen. She pressed a key and Bubbles' face appeared on the moonstone bead, she tapped another and Matilda's face appeared on the adjacent sapphire.

'I'm sure you do, you wicked woman. Do you know what time it is? His voice was deep and amused. Rosalie smiled. She wedged the 'phone between her shoulder and ear and curled herself like a cat into the armchair.

'Time we were in bed?'

Rosalie lifted the computer onto her lap and pressed a key. Bubbles' face faded into nothingness.

'Seriously though, I wondered if you were around tomorrow?'

'I think that could be arranged.'

'Matilda has to work, perhaps you'd like to show me some of the sights of this big ol' town ...?'

Finished! Must remember to return it to Undine.

****

Bubbles

Bubbles was lying on the bed in her room, the cockatiels were asleep under a striped flannelette sheet draped over their cage. She was deciphering one of her old scrawled diaries:

I don't have a home to go to. I wrote to Grania four months ago, soon after my seventeenth birthday, to ask if I could visit home one week-end a month and she wrote back saying No, not that often, I had my own home now.

After the big picture with broken glass slipped off the chair and almost decapitated Cal in his sleep, we had it re-glazed and now it hangs crookedly from a nail in the wall. The fireplace looked a lot better since I had removed the plywood panel covering. I was really excited by these improvements to my bedsit. The flimsy sash window still admitted whistling draughts which the 2-bar electric fire did little to combat, but visual excitement is always preferable to comfort. It was lucky that it did look aesthetically pleasing, as it gave Old Stover [mercenary landlord] less cause to complain. Someone is struggling frantically with the bathroom door, trying to lock it, the lock sticks sometimes - typical of everything in this old, badly-built house, obviously of the Ragged Trousered Philanthropist period. I shift my warm legs in bed. Outside the sun has risen and it looks as though it will be a sunny day, which always makes me feel depressed as it expects too much happiness in response. It's easier when it's grey, drizzling and undemanding. I can see an aeroplane humming across the sky; when it reaches a certain place on the window, the ripple of war glass causes the 'plane momentarily to switch course, before continuing onward. The sash window vibrates. The bath tap has been turned off, as all the pipes in the house stop hissing and judder for a couple of minutes instead. A cloud whisks across the sun, oh good, less pressure to go out in it and sunbathe. I could go and visit Helena today though. But no, her mother wheels glorious cream cakes into their suburban sitting-room at five o'clock on a trolley. If I relapse and partake of delicious comestibles my concave stomach will be convex when I see V playing in the band at the pub tonight. Just have enough money left for a face pack, will condition my hair for double the length of time it says to, and clean my teeth for five minutes with Baking Soda.

I'm sure it's Cal ringing. I sit tensely on the edge of my bed, looking at the blues of the cover I've made by doing as neat a running stitch as I can manage with double thickness thread, attaching a batique Indian bed cover to an old cotton sheet. This is to conceal my old thin sleeping bag, and transform it into a duvet. The 'phone is still ringing loudly and relentlessly, echoing against the walls of the communal hall. My step-mother always made a big fuss about making beds immaculately – 'You make your bed you lie in it.' I hope it's written on her tombstone. I wasn't allowed to make my own bed, ever, in case I didn't make it well enough. You can draw your own conclusions: it took me until now to have the strength of childhood conviction – what is the point of making a bed (except to save others' sensibilities) when you are only going to sleep in it again soon? It only needs to be left open to air so far as I'm concerned. I hear irate footsteps crashing against the stairs, the 'phone stops ringing. Is my privacy to be invaded this quiet sunny afternoon? 'I'm sure she's in, hold on,' the wall pay-phone receiver is dropped onto the wooden hall chest. Footsteps approach my door and a fist thumps on it. 'Phone for you! Would be good of you to answer it occasionally seeing as your door is nearest and it's always for you!' There's a silence: I sit, scarcely breathing. The footsteps go away.

Grey flapping billowing sky pinned like a grubby sheet to the towers around the Market Place. Twilight lent a pregnancy to the October sky and street lamps began to click into life. Walking home along the High Street towards Magdalen Bridge, looking up and watching the tops of the Oxford buildings like masts on a ship, scudding along beneath the dark clouds.

****

Gabriel

Boat Race Day was great, even though I wanted Cambridge to win, having done my degree there. It was very exciting jumping up and down on Big Girl's deck with me shouting 'Cambridge' and Torquil shrieking ' Oxford!' *The Ark* was chucked around on the wash from the Press launches like a bit of flotsam, but Gin just sat on the front doormat and washed himself. What a cool cat. And the new kitchen is coming along well. I think Torquil felt guilty about so summarily ripping out the old one, as he's been doing quite a lot of the work himself, along with his mate Robin. We found a Belfast sink in really good condition, dumped beside a skip in Acton. The things people chuck out!

****

Bubbles

Bubbles was fearfully skimming another diary:

I hit Cal first when I was 16, then he started hitting me back, soon it was just him hitting me. Once, when I was still living there, I went home with a black eye and William pointed it out to Grania at breakfast. I said hurriedly, oh no, it's where my eye makeup's run, it doesn't hurt. Grania just looked at me and didn't say anything. Once Cal threatened me in a doorway with a sliver of glass to my throat he'd grabbed off the pavement. I put my hand up and he accidentally cut my finger. I had to hold my fingers under a tap in the pub toilet for ages before the water ran clear. I was embarrassed and trying to hide the red flow swirling down the plughole. All round me, teenagers my age were excitedly and obliviously tarting themselves up in the mirrors. I wanted to keep seeing Cal as I didn't have anyone else. I was addicted to the relationship and I thought I deserved the violence. I'd been taught to endure, not to be a coward: there's a very fine line between that and masochism. Anyway my fears encroached too much to be at home much. By the end I was terrified of Cal, but I never really blamed him because he fell in love with me, and I'd bothered him constantly with my worries about whether I'd murdered a man who died. Cal couldn't cope; I spent all his money, soured his relations with his mother so that he had to move out (I spent so much time with him in his room at their house) plus I was often a right bitch. Grania was no keener on the relationship than his family, she being a rampant snob – so I wanted to see him all the more. For Cal's part, he resented me trying to better myself by doing evening classes, he was pleased when I initially failed my English A level (I was skiving classes to see him). He was a talented artist, but worked in a factory like his Dad. Cal's pet name for me was 'Moonshine'.

Ironically as soon as we had somewhere to go where we could spend all night together without the challenge of the deceit and adversity to see each other, the relationship folded. When I told him it was over, Cal was frighteningly upset and briefly violent, but forcibly restrained by some of my new friends as I stood rigid and terrified in the street. As Joanna and Emma held onto his arms - they were much braver than their scared boyfriends - Cal suddenly collapsed into noisy tears and said sobbing: 'I don't understand Moonshine, I haven't hit you for a week, why are you finishing it now? We'll get married if you like.'

****

Bubbles

Unfortunately I had a deep chat with Chloris after returning home early from the pub. I was feeling too tense amongst the crowds to stay any longer. I kept visualising that I'd dropped broken glass into someone's drink. When I left, I only managed to get out by following the wall round to the door, trying not to touch it or anyone. I did look back several times, checking that I hadn't harmed anyone, then a guy saw me doing it and gave me a strange look. I felt awful, utterly conspicuous. When I finally got outside the pub, I had a panic attack about leaving marks with my heels on the pavement and thought I was going to cry. I didn't tell Chloris any of this, of course; in fact I was flippant. Well, until she began lecturing me horribly about my character, social flaws, Marius' faults, etcetera. I suppose I might like a fascinating job, but there's not much hope of me finding that as, apart from writing, drawing and travelling, I don't know what I want to do. Also, I still haven't sorted out the contradictory thoughts in my head about earning money when I have strong socialist ideals. I'm desperate for success, but I'm scared of it too.

Chloris hasn't emptied the bin, again! I noticed this when she was in full spate, but didn't know how to say anything about it in a way I'd be happy with afterwards. Anyway, it's so anal to bother about housework, I hate the way I'm so fastidious, despite all my home-made aversion therapy. I need lessons in assertiveness: so that I can say what I really mean, particularly when someone is being unfair or upsets me – like Alex stopping the session early.

Think I'll move out.

****

Romance

Ursula could hear odd sentences from her friends' conversation in the sitting-room: 'We'll get married at the Register Office next month' said Ali excitedly.
'Ursula'll have to move all her clothes and things in your bedroom for the visit by the authorities, or do they just interview you both in an office?' she heard Fatima ask. Ali's reply was inaudible.
To Ursula's relief when she went upstairs, she discovered the flat had three large bedrooms. Ali's was decorated in maroon and dark green; further along the passage was a slightly smaller room, sunnily painted yellow with an en-suite bathroom. She wondered if she could use that, as the third room seemed to be Ali's home office complete with a roll-top desk, and computer. She was struck by the absence of papers on show, not even computer disks. On impulse Ursula tried a desk drawer, it was locked.
'I'm off now Ursula' called Fatima, making her jump. Feeling ashamed of herself, Ursula hurried out of the study.
'I'll come too'. She arranged with Ali that they would speak on the phone affectionately and daily, to get into the habit and in case phone bills were later scanned by the authorities. 'I shall enjoy it' said Ali gallantly. Ursula thought to herself that she would find it more difficult.

As she and Fatima chatted on the way to the Knightsbridge tube station, she was daunted by the amount of things she would need to know about Ali. His favourite colours, foods, habits, all about his childhood, family history, the names of his relatives. At least all his family lived abroad, apart from one brother who lived in Manchester. This made things much easier. Ursula didn't know if she could have coped with the deception involved in being a loving daughter-in-law.

The next day Ursula rang Sarah to tell her she was moving. Sarah plied her with questions.
'I'm moving into a shared flat' Ursula improvised quickly. She had visions of Ali answering the phone to her friends: 'He's an old friend' she added uncomfortably.
'Oh, really?' Sarah was intrigued.
Ursula felt guilty: it was her first experience of serious deception. Sarah was impressed by Ursula's new address: 'That's really close to Harrods, isn't it? How much is the rent - do you don't mind me asking?' Ursula made up a ridiculously low amount, then pointed out quickly that the old friend owned it. The more questions she fielded, the more tangled she felt in her web of deceit. She had to fight the urge to tell her friend about her impending marriage. Sarah unknowingly heaped coals on Ursula's head, by indignantly refusing the extra rent money Ursula offered in lieu of notice.
'You must come over sometime.'
Ursula agreed rather desperately, trying to avoid a solid arrangement, and rang off with relief.

The following week, Ali collected Ursula with her possessions packed into boxes and bags, in his new white convertible Mercedes. They had to make two trips
between Kensington and Knightsbridge to move everything. Ursula felt a sudden sharp pang at leaving her old flat; she stood alone in the spotless sunny sitting-room, empty now of her pictures and books, and looked around. She had been very happy there - until Anthony had appeared in her life with such devastating consequences. Her treacherous thoughts reminded her of the expression in his eyes when he had walked in on her after her bath.
Then of watching him disappear through the front door. This bleak memory cancelled a strong temptation to call off the

arrangement with Ali. With a deep sigh Ursula walked along the hall, picking up a last bag of things on the way. She carefully locked the front door behind her, putting the bag down to post her set of keys through the newly repaired letter box as arranged. Ali hooted impatiently from the packed car downstairs; Ursula tried to ignore the way his face lit up as he saw her close the front door and hurry down the steps.

Ali started the engine, and turned up a CD of the Rolling Stones. He gently drummed his fingers on the steering wheel in time to the music. 'Is that everything Ursula?' 'Yes, thank you': she craned round to look back at the windows of her old home, receding into the distance. Ali expertly accelerated into the busy traffic flowing towards Knightsbridge: the die was well and truly cast.

****

Three months after their quiet wedding, Ursula couldn't believe how well things had worked out. As she had anticipated, Ali had not immediately accepted that theirs was to be a purely platonic relationship. When he insisted on buying Ursula a 24ct platignum wedding ring studded with diamonds, she looked at him apprehensively. 'But Ali, this is much too expensive." she exclaimed. 'What if I lose it?' 'It doesn't matter' he said grandly. 'No wife of mine is going to want.' Then he grinned reassuringly at her worried face. He had tried to take Ursula romantically into his arms after an evening out, during the first week, but following a firm rebuff had regretfully toed the line. Ursula was surprised by how considerate Ali had turned out to be. He hid his longing for her, if that's what it was - she sometimes felt it was all a macho act - under outrageous compliments which made her laugh.

Even the interview with the authorities had gone smoothly. Ursula had felt revulsion as she forced herself to act the part of a loving wife, but it seemed to convince the humourless officials. One of them had even offered congratulations. Ursula reflected she obviously wasn't cut out to be a criminal - breaking the law made her feel dreadful. She would give anything now to be clear of this 'marriage' but she had entered a contract. It was part of her personal creed to abide by promises; this was why she felt she had had to continue sending her parents money. She had said to Ali she would stay a year, so a year it had to be. Ursula consoled herself slightly with the thought that a quarter of the time had already passed.

This crisp autumnal morning Ursula reflected, she and Ali appeared the picture of friendly domesticity. While she busily made toast and grilled bacon, Ali sat at the breakfast table buried in the newspaper. 'How many pieces of toast, Ali?' She looked over his shoulder: as usual he was reading the racing results. He was obsessed with his racehorse, Pride and Prejudice.
'Ali?' she prompted.
'Two, please' he muttered absently. He jerked his head up: 'Ursula, you don't have to make breakfast for me'.
'I know, but I enjoy cooking'. A yearning expression crossed his face: 'No Ali, I enjoy cooking equally for anyone', she said firmly. 'Oh,' he pretended great disappointment. 'Pride and Prejudice should be ready to race at Kempton next Spring Ursula, he's coming on well.' He put the newspaper aside with a rustle as she set a full plate before him. 'This looks delicious, thanks'. Ursula sat down with her plate and waited for the usual plea: 30 seconds, 50 seconds, one minute then-
'Ursula how about going shopping for some clothes?'
'Ali you are so predictable!'
'I insist on lending you the money, if you're still sure you won't let me buy you anything' he pleaded. 'Come on Ursula, you only live once.'
'Oh, all right' she finally capitulated.
'Great! Finish your breakfast and I'll take the car. We'll go to Josephs, Selfridges, Browns-'
'Hey, calm down Ali. Listen to this,' she said teasingly '...I thought I might go the whole way and have my hair seen to as well. How's that?'

He was thrilled. At times like this, she thought, he was like a pleasant younger brother - although she was actually the younger by five years. He increased her confidence, and it was fun living with someone who enjoyed life so much. She found herself wishing again that she could fall in love with Ali, it would make life so easy. Instead of which, she often had to push unwelcome memories of Anthony's tall dark good looks from her mind. The way his fingers slid slowly through her hair when she was caught against him, trying to make her dramatic exit from 'Clouds'. Ursula cringed inwardly.

****

Bubbles

This therapy is like struggling through a huge thorn hedge with no visible way out. I just know I can't go back, or stop. I'm in terrible pain sometimes.

I sat on the edge of a Gothic defunct Church pew in the hall of the mansion in Eaton Place.
 I could hear Ax and his previous client, who had over-run his hour. The guy sounded about my age and surprisingly cheerful.
'So when can you make it?'
'How about Monday the 26th?'
'Yes, fine. Urmm, oh, no sorry, I already have someone booked in then. '
Pause, rattle of pages
'I can do Tuesday the 27th'
'Yes, that looks all right.... How about six o'clock?'
I inspected the parquet flooring and my boots resting theron. My link to the Earth.
'Oh, no, I don't finish work until five-thirty and then-'
Friday the 30th?'
'Yes, sure.'
'Oh that's good. Would you be able to come at lunchtime?'
I shifted centimetre by centimetre into a slightly more relaxed position on the chair, and surveyed the large Arabic glass lamps suspended from the centre of the white panelled ceiling.
'Well... It might be a struggle to get from EC2 to here though and back in time, though the scooter's good... Maybe I could.'
'Oh no, you don't want to jeopardize the Inkblot job,'
Conspiratorial laughter.

The hall is vast, the row of lamps diminishes into the distance towards the monumental wooden front door with stained glass panels. I stared down at my hands painfully clamped together so that the flesh shone white. Eventually I forced myself to look at the pen lying on brass tray on the marble table next to me. It was a wooden pencil, lying bathed in the peaceful light of a desk lamp. Had I touched it?

'Well how about Wednesday 5th as Tuesday's so difficult?'

'You know, I could do that – oh hang on, I think Kathy has arranged something for that night.'

My hands hurt: I wondered if I'd lifted the pencil, and written something untrue about my brother on the wallpaper. The message would be found by someone else, who would publicise it.

'Perhaps we need to speak on the 'phone, when you have your diary in front of you..?'

Then the terrifying people would find out and whatever happened to me, everyone would think I deserved it, particularly me. I realised I was holding my breath and with difficulty forced myself to exhale. I listened carefully to the breath in case there were any words in it.

'Yeah, I'm a bit hard to get hold of… What about Friday 7th?'

I breathed in carefully. My heart beat painfully hard, I bit my tongue. I hadn't said anything while caught in the tornado of thoughts, had I?

'I'm off to Belgium that day, sorry,'

'No', I exclaimed aloud, to negate anything I might have said, and clamped my tongue between my teeth again. I was burning hot, my tongue ached. I wanted to take my coat off, but was too scared of dropping something on the floor.

Grania had snapped: 'Hold your tongue!' I remembered sitting on the low chair in the kitchen, listening to 'Children's Hour' on the old-fashioned radio on the red painted shelf high up on the white wall above the mangle. My toes just touched the quarry tiles. Grania was eating at the kitchen table next to me, a book propped up against a milk bottle in front of her. I tried to comprehend what Grania meant, I held my tongue with my fingers. I didn't understand what she was doing, staring silently at the pages. The enamelled stove door in front of me was cream-coloured, with a black iron handle.

'I tell you what, why don't you ring me when you have your diary in front of you?' Ax was still sounding relaxed and courteous. With the small part of my mind still looking outward, I was impressed.

Had I spelt out anything with my brown leather boots touching the parquet floor? I craned down, head between my knees, to see. The sitting room door opened, I sat upright reluctantly. There was a mark on the honey-coloured wood, did it spell anything? It looked a bit like an 'M', which could denote 'murder'. I tapped the floor twice with my toe to indicate the letters N.O.

Ax hurried out saying: 'Let me just get those for you,' he scooped up a jacket and bag from a chair in the hall, and exited stage right.

I sat upright; I could check the floor again when I stood up. I'd need to look at the pencil and table too. Suddenly there were people emerging from the consulting room on the right of the hall. I tried to breathe deeply but the air stopped at the bottom of my throat. Distantly I smiled in response, as Ax beamed at me briefly. He escorted the patient, disguised by crash helmet and swaddled in black leather, to the door. He shook hands with him.

'I'll call you.'

'Great, have a good week,' said Alex, watching him descend the steps.

****

Alexander

'Hi, come in.' Alexander wondered in passing why Undine was flushed. She was always swathed in layers, he suspected against him and his probing questions. He wondered if she still had an eating disorder. Despite her breezy assertion that she'd recovered, she looked skinny. 'Would you like to take off your coat?' That was one way of checking whether she was emaciated.

'No, thanks.' She pulled it round herself and looked at the seat carefully before sitting down.

Oh hell, I forgot to ring Wendy back and I won't have time later. She's getting a bit intense which is a drag. Lucy and I

have just been invited to a concert at the Barbican, we're in a private box with Lord and Lady Effluent. Fantastic!.
'Er, I'm awfully sorry Undine, but I need to urgently call a patient. I have to cancel an appointment, they're in rather a state.'
I think Undine said 'So am I,' but it was said very quietly.
When I looked at her enquiringly, she said politely: 'Go ahead, I don't mind what you do in sessions, within reason'.
'We'll go on for longer at the end, of course,' I smiled at her warmly before popping out into the hall with the mobile.

****

Bubbles

I could hear bits of the conversation:
'Of course, me too.'
'I'm sorry but it can't be helped, Lucy didn't tell me until-'
Just as I was beginning to twitch again, although it was probably no longer than a couple of minutes, I heard Ax say distinctly, 'You're being tiresome Wendy!' It made my nerves jump: I hope he doesn't ever speak to me like that.

Ax was back, looking bland, but with a faint sheen of perspiration on his upper lip. He must have unobstrusively wiped it off, because it wasn't there next time I looked across at him.
'I have a couple of things I really want to achieve,' I gabbled. This was safe territory and might keep us away from distressing areas. 'Just side products. One is to grow my hair: I've done everything with it, dyed it every colour you can imagine, shaved it off, permed it, had long hair extensions put in - I've even had long black dreadlocks. My step-mother had very long hair and I wasn't allowed to grow mine.'
'I don't think you need permission from me really.'
Permission: what an interesting idea.
'I also want to get down a Red Run.' Heaven knows when I'll be able to afford to go to the mountains again, but that's neither here nor there.
'Is that ski-ing?' he asked, to my surprise, I'd assumed it went with his lifestyle. Although actually, I realised, I didn't know much about Ax's life at all.

Yes, it's a steep slope.'
His face lit up, 'Do you suffer from vertigo?'
'Yes, but it's getting better.'
'Have you tried the Whispering Gallery at St. Paul's?'
'Yes, I just clung to the wall, walked a few steps along then had to go down. It took two hours once to get me down some outside steps in Turkey. I was like one of those toys with suckers that people stick onto car windows, I had to be prized off every step.'
He nodded, knowingly.
'I'm fine going up, it's coming down.' Good analogy for drugs. Maybe I can work it so that Ax and I go out somewhere public together, maybe a dry ski slope …

Ax tried to steer the conversation back to me recording my anxiety levels, when checking whether taps, the iron and the stove were turned off. The sort of thing many people worry about, but don't keep returning to stare at so that they're late for everything. On very bad, mercifully rare, days, I don't get out at all. I managed to distract Ax by telling him funny stories about when I hitch-hiked round Europe and begged in Italy, four years ago.

It was almost time to go, I am good at calculating time in my head.
'Logs,' he said.
I had a vision of a raft on the river, rough wood full of integrity, floating and turning at the beck of the current, borne up by the maelstrom beneath.
'Here,' Ax said, pulling out a piece of paper from a pile on the table. It was a pre-printed hospital 'history sheet' with spaces for unit numbers, names, dates and clinical notes on it.
'I'll just put washing machine being off … taps… ' He wrote a neat list.
'Oh damn, I thought I'd done a good job of distracting you, Alexander,' I said.
'What are the other things that you're finding difficult on the checking front at the moment, Undine?'
The empty raft floated away.
'Um, not closing the cat in the door, making sure that the iron is off.' Prickly tears were surfacing.

'Right, I've put those down. Now the dates across the top. Each day I want you during one of the checking occasions – not every time otherwise it gets a bit silly – to write down your anxiety level out of ten. Ten is absolutely the worst you can feel.'
'Ten is the worst...' I was trying to understand how it works.
'How do you feel at the moment?'
'About five?' I was beginning to bite my tongue and my hands were clenched in my pockets. 'Shall we put down more categories?' I asked with difficulty, releasing my tongue briefly.
'We don't want too many, we could do it all quickly, but the effect won't last. This does work.'
I managed to unclench my hand out of my pocket, looked at my finger tips to check for marks, then disbelievingly took the proffered sheet.

I had a hangover again. I was beginning to realise that I binge drank at a small bar in Holborn at least twice a week, because I always had a sick headache and couldn't remember much about the previous night when I attended my new Saturday morning tuition. Amazingly I'd won a course of ten driving lessons in a raffle at the Wine Bar.
'There's a pigeon over there!' I said nervously, looking ahead at a concrete courtyard inside a Council estate.
'Never mind the pigeon, it's miles away! Watch the parked cars, you're too close. See that woman? She looks as though she's going to cross, she hasn't heard you.'
I rammed my foot on the brake. 'Did I run her over?'
'No, you were nowhere near her. Now, mirror, signal, manoevre. Mirror, signal ... Undine, mirror!'
Phil stamped on the brake, and we jerked to an emergency stop behind a lorry.
'I was going to pull out.'
'We would have hit that bollard! Do as I say, when I say it.'
Phil's relaxed attitude and arm hanging negligently out of the car window were a thing of the past. He breathed deeply in the silence for a moment or two.

'Let's try again. Don't forget, foot off clutch gently, Undine, gently!' We stalled.

At the next attempt to drive off, I stared round so paranoically at the blind spot that I got a crick in my neck and it took us five minutes to move at all.

'Now indicate, we are going left, ' intoned Phil with forced patience. The indicator ticked. 'Good. Into second gear and round the corner, while the lights are green.'

I pulled the lever around firmly, we reversed, at speed.

'Christ!'

I screamed and took both hands off the wheel. There was a sound of smashing glass and a grating along Phil's side of the car. He put his foot on the brake, and wrenched the steering wheel round. He stared in his mirror before opening the door. 'That's the first time that's happened to me in nine years!' he said, he seemed stunned. He was gone for ages, trying to find the owner of the shiny Audi sports car. I sat clutching my hands, trying not to panic. I could just see at an angle through the side window how the Audi wing mirror made an attractive floor mosaic.

****

Gabriel

I suddenly realised that Florence and Maisie were holding onto the desk, crying with laughter. Panting, I dragged back the wheelchair housing the overweight patient and doggedly tried to steer it round another low armchair in Reception. The waiting area was a veritable obstacle course and Pam Webb very heavy. The hospital porter had slunk off, probably for a cigarette, so I was trying to help out.

'Where are the brakes on this thing?' I asked, clinging onto the chair as we shot forward and bashed into a low table.

'I can walk,' squawked the patient in panic, trying to rise. Fortunately she seemed to be wedged in place.

'No,' I said determinedly, I refused to be out-manoevred by a wheelchair. 'You're entitled to a lift. We'll get you to the Scanning Room.'

I was sweating by the time we reached the swing doors, the smooth linoleum was even harder to steer on than carpet. The heavy swing doors seemed to be stuck. I shoved them again hard, this time with my shoulder. Pam shrieked as the wheelchair swivelled in a frivolous *pas de deux*. Fluorescent lighting reflected off the grey shining floor. She was trying to get out of her chair again, an impatient patient, some people don't know when they're well off. I was exhausted and would have welcomed someone wheeling me around. I placed a soothing hand on Pam's plump shoulder.

'Lemme get off,' she yelled, pulling at the blanket across her knees. I wondered if Lazarus had been this annoying. Perhaps Christ had been trying to invent a wheelchair then given up: Oh all right, take up your bed and walk then!

'Not far now, I said with false bonhomie, wishing Maisie would come and help.

'Gabriel,' she was beside me. 'There's someone trying to get through from the other side.'

She giggled, even Pam smiled.

Sure enough, through the narrow pane of glass in the door, I saw an irate porter pushing at the door and saying something succinct to his patient in a wheelchair who was looking smug.

'I can walk!' Pam's pink blanket fell to the floor and got caught under the wheel.

'Okay,' I said, giving up the struggle. I pulled back the chair with difficulty, at which point the swing doors banged open and the oncoming vehicle ran over my foot.

There's one consolation, at least I'm not as hopeless at this job as Torquil would be. I had gastric 'flu once, which I wouldn't wish on my worst enemy, and Torquil promptly moved out for a week, saying I was no fun. Torquil will have to promise never to come near me if I'm terminally ill - he probably wouldn't anyway, in case he caught it.

There was the time when Don James, who lives on a trawler further out in the river, said: 'Of course I'm very poorly, all down here.' He undid his trousers before our horrified eyes and pulled down one side, exposing pallid plump flesh reminiscent of the white slugs found in undisturbed dark places. He pointed to an otherwise healthy-looking leg.

'I'll die soon,' he added pathetically shuffling to an armchair and sitting down jerkily with a grunt. His daughter looked concerned and as though she'd like to shut him up.

'Oh well, comes to us all!' said Torquil cheerfully, looking at his watch.

Everyone in the room looked tensely at Mr. James, the lines of whose face suddenly rearranged themselves into a delighted smile.

'Well, I suppose so.' he said. 'What did you say your name was again, young man?'

Cemeteries are listed under Council 'Leisure Services' in the 'phone book. Torquil can't decide where he wants to be buried, it changes from week to week. I'd drop his corpse over the side, but he'd revisit *The Ark* every time the tide came in.

Maybe I could make transparent water beds with fish inside, or transparent baths with fish swimming inside the walls? It would be too mean for the fish with the bed idea though, too many waves. Anyway, how would they censor what young fish saw before the 9pm watershed?

Get on with some work Gabriel! I must remember to pick up cat comestibles and human food on the way home, from Hammersmith, oh and a copy of *The Stage*. I'm losing focus.

****

Bubbles

The diaries were open:

I was terrified that Simon would hit me, in retrospect without justification. I bleakly held the view that the world is run on the premise that men are physically stronger than women. Now I have an understanding that brains or cunning are behind true power, although they often utilise brutality. Emotional coercion of that sort seems to be almost as prevalent among women as men. Interrogation of Simon was typical in form of seeking reassurance, which of course another human being can scarcely ever bestow. Faith is involved, and while I appeared to trust everybody, getting into all sorts of bizarre situations, actually I didn't trust anybody – least of all myself:

'Would you ever hit me?
'No'

Did you say Yes or No?
'No'
'What, you didn't say No?'
'No, I said Yes - I mean No.'
'You said 'Yes' Simon, that means you'll hit me.'
'I didn't mean that I would hit you.'
'But you said you would.'
'No, I didn't.'
Yes you did, you said "Yes".'

'I meant to say "No"'.

'What did you say?'
'I said, I meant to say "'No"'.'
'Can you repeat that?'
'I said, I meant to say "No" .'
'So you wouldn't hit me..?'
'No!'
'Did I make you say that? And, no, you wouldn't hit me, or you wouldn't not?'

And so on, and on, for hours of dread, sweat and fear. Living through others is dangerous: you float or shatter with every word.

She had a big hole where her Self should be. She tried unsuccessfully to fill this with sex, thought, dreams, food, alcohol, drugs, oblivion. One drop of loving compassion from Grania would have filled and healed the ulcerous wound.

I used to mascara my eyelashes, apply foundation, blusher and lipstick - have a full glamorous facemask before I'd emerge into the Oxford day. I used to hide in doorways, thinking I was ugly, scared to look at people. People used to complain that I ignored them, but I never saw them.

You stop smelling after about six weeks if you don't wash, then scrape down with sand or mud – I know that from later on, doing my own aversion therapy to cleanliness, and demonstrating to stop them chopping down trees to build motorways. I handcuffed myself to a large lump of concrete underground. People thought I was brave, but I was reckless because I thought I was immortal and didn't give a shit what happened to me anyway.

'8st.3lbs, lose 7 lbs before I see Paul on Sunday! He called me 'Thunderthighs' last week and Cal laughed. I'll get a load of speed off Johnny.

Calories: 1800 so far today, all right if I stop eating now (11am) until tomorrow morning. Did 40 sit-ups and walked ten miles yesterday out to Kidlington and back.

However thin I get, my hip bones are still wider than my waist, how thin do you get before there's only the skeleton? You could plane off bone then, to have boyish hips. I am so ugly, I try and squeeze my spots at night - getting rid of the impurity feels so rewarding - so that I'm not too blotchy the next day and can't go outside. I avoid mirrors completely otherwise, so that I don't see the blemishes. I scrub my face, neck, back and shoulders sometimes, with a nail brush and soap, to make the spots go away. I wish I wasn't so pale but I never have enough money in one go to escape, to travel to sunshine.

Grania's letting William store stuff at home since he moved out, she never would have let me. She's lent him money. He's not her child, any more than I am, why does she treat us so differently? It must be my fault.

I can't help it; I go to the wardrobe and, crouching down, lift up the heavy door. I wriggle half-way underneath and pull out the full packet of cracker biscuits, butter and half a pound of cheese-.

Bubbles slammed the diary shut and hurled it back into the cardboard box.

....

Bubbles had been to pay tribute to Marx's tomb at Highgate Cemetery; a man from the Council was cleaning graffiti off it again with white spirit. Now she sat on a bench in Waterlow Park. She threw a crust to an aggressive squirrel which stood on its hind legs a few feet away, chittering at her. It turned the bread busily in it's paws as it munched, the breeze ruffled it's delicate, bushy tail. Branches of trees clicked together in the chilly breeze. Bubbles pulled her bent notepad and a pen clumsily from her jacket pocket. She propped her heel on the bench and opened the book, resting it on her bent knee.

She looked with disbelief: someone had been reading her Romance. The pages were grimy; at the end of her last sentence, a stranger had clumsily scrawled in red pen: 'They fucked under water! The End.' Someone else had written 'load of crap' in tiny, lethal, blue letters. Bubbles sat on in shock, the wind moving her hair. She didn't recognise the writing, it wasn't Marius's and he was the only one who might have found the book in her room. Where had she left the notebook when she'd carried it up there a few days ago? She'd found it on the mantelpiece just now. Bubbles tried to breathe evenly but her heart hammered. She realised gradually that she was getting cold. She slowly closed the book and replaced it in her pocket, then stood looking at the empty wooden bench for a couple of minutes. Turning away with an effort, she blew on her fingers and walked along the path towards Swains Lane. The squirrel followed.

****

Marius

Stupid tarts, I only left them alone while I took a slash. I've had to listen to Bubbles all morning, going on and on about her stupid story. I did point out that it was my notebook, hinting that she shouldn't have nicked it. She eventually bought the idea that whoever had written silly remarks on it might think they were insulting my 'art' rather than hers, as my name's still in small letters on the cover. When she's wound up like that though, it takes ages to soothe her into a receptive enough state for me to satisfy my nasty carnal desires, so I got pissed off. I'll have to be more careful, I'm used to getting the frost treatment from Witch Chloris, but Matilda's joined the coven now. I was sure they were out when I brought Fi and Sam round. I tiptoed round the house listening at doors before I let them in, giggling, over the threshold.

I keep the stuff in Bubbles's room, in the pockets of my shirt hanging from the picture rail. People don't think to look at what's right under their nose. Can't keep the gear at my gaff at the moment, had the Filth round only last month, Vince tipped me off they were coming. It almost got out of control yesterday in Bubbles' bedroom, I wasn't quite myself - nor were Sam and Fi once they'd tried the merchandise. As soon as I'd realised Bubbles was out, the temptation to have a bit of fun with the girls was overwhelming. Lucky I heard that door slam, I got us dressed and out of there just in time.

****

Bubbles

I'm being deafened by a loud siren; instantly I'm awake. The siren is one of the cockatiels scolding the other, clambering busily across the bars of the metal cage. The front door slams, far below. I carefully open my eyes. A thin laser of dazzling sunlight shoots below the dusty sheet spread across the window, and stripes the floorboards. I'm alive, I'm here, right now. I turn my body carefully beneath the rough grey blanket and peer at the floor beside the bed. I can see a gin bottle, empty, next to it an ashtray full of cigarette ends and a bottle top. Can I sit up? I try, and the blanket falls back to show yesterday's clothes. My legs are encased in laddered stockings and short, twisted, red skirt, comfortable though. My limbs feel bruised, my mouth feels horrible. I can smell stale alcohol. I feel my hair, matted, there's something encrusted at the back. I stare at the dark grit under my fingernails, it looks like dried blood. I can't smell anything horrible on my hands, although they're black with filth. It's heavenly sitting here, thinking nothing, relaxed. I'm remembering bits now. I drank the bottle of gin last night to numb the pain, it must have worked because nothing matters now. I'm glad to be here, released briefly from anxiety into another day. How wonderful that day follows night.

....

After a relaxing bath, Bubbles wandered, light-footed, into the kitchen, Matilda looked at her strangely, halting toast half-way to her mouth. 'There's some coffee left if you want some? Over there.'

'Oh, thanks.'

Bubbles sank down into a chair, putting her cup on the table, and smiled across at Matilda. She felt cleansed and relaxed. 'God, I was wrecked last night.'

'I know,' said Matilda, looking thoughtfully down at her plate. 'Do you remember anything?'

'Well, I remember ... No, I don't really.'

'Not the Police bringing you home?'

'The Police!' Bubbles's stomach melted with horror. 'I don't remember that at all. What did I say to them? What happened? '

Apparently you threw a drink all over a friend of Vivienne's in the 'Horse and Groom' at Hampstead, you kicked another woman really hard. Marius was with you, but it sounds as though he just left you, the bastard.'

'I don't know, it was probably my fault. Vivienne was there?' Bubbles felt chilled with fear. She was remembering fragments now, of stamping along a lamp-lit pavement, screaming abuse after the dark flickering figure hurrying away. 'I smashed a bottle of wine in the street, in the middle of Hampstead, I remember lights coming on in windows. That was after the pub though, I think. It must have been.'

'They were probably the ones who called the Police.'

'Was the woman, the women, in the pub, all right?'

'I guess so, the police didn't say anything other than what I've told you. Nobody's pressing charges that I know of.'

'And they brought me back here?'

'After you'd thrown up over a policewoman's arm. You're lucky they brought you home after all that.'

'I remember keep trying to ring Marius from a call box and getting the wrong number. The man was livid, he said it was four o'clock and I didn't understand what he was on about ...'

'Bubbles, you can't go on like this. Chloris persuaded the plods to leave you here and calmed everyone down.'

'Chloris!' All Bubbles' ideas of independence and being able to hold her drink, slid sideways.

As if on cue, Chloris appeared in the doorway, she seemed to be in a hurry.

'Morning Undine.'

'Um, thanks, I've just heard that you stood up for me last night.'

'It's all right. I suppose. How often are you getting blotto like that?'

'I don't know, say once or twice a week? But I don't have to have a drink every day, so I'm not an alcoholic.'

'There's such a thing as a binge alcoholic Undine. I've just never seen the rest of your evening arriving home with you.'

'Except for too many strange guys,' interjected Matilda,

'But that hasn't been for a while,' asked Bubbles anxiously.

'Well, not for a few months, since you and Marius got back together.'

....

Today, there was an oriental man standing playing the violin in the Mall, amidst the indifferent lunchtime throng of workers and school adolescents. I was really glad of soothing music, after the shock yesterday of hearing what I'd done when inebriated. No Bubbles, pissed out of your brains, grasp the nettle. Nearby a tall gangly chap, leaning against a pink tiled wall, was listening to the violinist with a beatific smile. Today the jerky man wasn't holding a beer can, as when he wandered anxiously past me last week, on his way to the Off Licence in Fulham Palace Road. I've seen Ali who runs it, here at the Mall. He's a middle-aged polite Indian man, with dark pouches of flesh under his eyes. He's kind to the scruffy alcoholics who gather outside his shop at opening time. Maria told me, she usually sits against the wall begging near the 'Metro' stand. She's got three kids, but she doesn't know where two of them are now.

The musician, who was dressed in black, had a quiet dignity. The bottom of his violin case, lying open on the ground, was almost concealed by coins of small denomination. The music he created was beautiful, it cut calmly through the turbulent air, making order from chaos. Speaking of beauty, I briefly noticed this very attractive tall guy, white-blond hair, striding out of Costalot-Caff wearing a long coat. I think he looked at me too – thank heaven for the gold paint.

I watched a young woman with light-brown hair; I felt sorry for her, she would have been really attractive if her face hadn't been so drawn. She kept inspecting a piece of blank white paper, turning it over. She held the paper up to the light, her lips were compressed like the Queen's, I saw her move her fingernails fiercely across it. Eventually she crumpled up the page and shoved it fiercely into her coat pocket. Then she took her hand out of her pocket slowly and inspected it carefully back and front. She sniffed it, frowning, several times. I noticed that the musician was watching her discreetly but kindly while he played. Then I observed this dark-haired plump woman staring spitefully. When the young woman saw her, the fat woman tapped her head meaningfully and laughed at her. The neurotic woman looked devastated. I wish now I'd said something comforting to her, and to hell with being statuesque. I probably look like her when I'm carrying out one of my checking rituals.

....

I saw the blonde man in the long coat in the supermarket after work. I was wandering along the isles with less need to check things than usual, perhaps because the shop was unusually deserted and I'd had a good night's sleep. I just received a vague impression of someone very tall with high cheekbones, perhaps with green eyes. Not my usual type, but the air was suddenly foggy with pheromones. It's the first time I've fancied anyone, apart from Ax, in a long time. I quickly shut my mind and sheered off along another aisle, swinging my basket. I stopped to indecisively regard the Bakery special offers, '8 for the price of 6', and became aware that *he* was standing beside me. So there we were, considering crumpet. I turned quickly to leave and a pleasant voice said: 'Excuse me, I know this is a strange question-'
I looked up at him quickly.
'But are you the living statue, who stands over there?' he asked in a rush, gesturing towards my empty dais which could be seen through the shop window.
'Er, yes.' He was speaking to *me.* His teeth were very white.

'Are you an actor?'

'Oh no.'

He had a lively, open expression. 'It's just that... Acting friends of mine occasionally do jobs like that between parts.'

'No, I'm a writer.' I said daringly.

He didn't laugh or look incredulous. 'Great, what sort of stuff do you do?' There are freckles across the bridge of his large beaky nose.

'Oh... All different things. Do you like the violin music?'

'Yes, isn't he fantastic? Oh, I'm Gabriel by the way,' he held out his hand.

'Bubbles,' I said laughing, shaking hands quickly. His palm was dry and warm.

We were off, talking all the way to the till queue and through it, so that I forgot to check whether I'd touched the conveyor belt in strange ways, or left anything under the spare plastic bags on the other side. The supermarket felt friendly and human, and not an overwhelming brightly-lit hell of alienation.

Gabriel's an actor; he's given me his mobile telephone number. He says he's having a land-line installed soon on the boat where he lives, which sounds odd. He's given me his e-mail too, but I haven't got my head round using internet cafés yet. I'd be too scared of the temptation to write something terrible about child abuse or something. Apparently Gabriel's vessel is moored at somewhere called Chiswick, two or three miles from here. I'm not able to use 'phones very well at the moment, I wonder if Matilda would let me borrow her mobile and show me how to text him? I feel sorry for Gabriel, stuck out in a west London suburb: central London's far more edgy and exciting. I noticed he limps too, poor thing.

****

Romance

Bubbles propped open her bedroom door, then pulled the chair up to her new table. Marius and Art had placed it in her room as a surprise, they didn't have room for the table at Art's place any more. Marius had been really kind lately, for which

Bubbles was grateful. She opened a new notebook and reached for the pen.

Ali pushed Ursula gently through the doorway of Moi; the hairdressing salon appeared intimidatingly grand from the outside, the assistants were dauntingly chic. Ursula stood mutely by the desk.
'Hi, oh hello' said a slim stylish man, recognising Ali. 'Not me today Crispin' said Ali quickly 'My wife is having her hair cut.' Ursula looked startled, then smiled apologetically. She still had problems remembering her role.
'You rang earlier, didn't you? Sue will be doing it - you have beautiful hair' he said appreciatively, looking at Ursula's hair pulled tightly back into a long plait.
'Thanks' muttered Ursula shyly.
'I'll meet you at the coffee bar we passed further along, say in an hour?' said Ali. 'I have to see to some business'. Ursula found herself wishing he wouldn't go. She felt conspicuous.
'Would you like to put on this robe?' a young woman held it outstretched, with a friendly smile.
Ursula watched Sue in the mirror expertly brush her hair. 'It's a lovely silvery colour, it's natural isn't it?' Ursula nodded. 'Right down to the bottom of your back' marvelled Sue. One of the other hairdressers looked across: 'We hardly ever get anyone in with hair as long as yours.'
'When did you last have it cut?' asked Sue.

'Well I trimmed it with the kitchen scissors a couple of weeks ago, but they're a bit blunt' said Ursula unthinkingly. She met Sue's horrified eyes in the mirror, and they both laughed: 'Not any more!' said Sue firmly. They decided Sue would cut a feathery fringe into the front of the heavy hair and up to two inches from the ends of the rest, so it was the same length all the way round. Later, after blow-drying Ursula's hair until it was a shining mane, Sue showed her how to roll it into a smooth French pleat. 'That's if you're going out somewhere smart, and want a change.' Ursula knew approximately how much the bill was going to be, but was still startled. 'Never mind' she thought firmly, adding a tip, 'This is the first time I've been to the hairdressers in years, and it's money I would have

spent on rent.' The manager suddenly said: 'Excuse me, would you mind if we took a photograph of you for our window?'
By the time Ursula met Ali she was feeling wonderful. He wolf-whistled as she ran across the street to the cafe to where he was seated outside in rather chilly sunshine. 'You look great!' he said standing up and staring admiringly. 'Do a twirl.' Ursula did, laughing, her hair swung round her like pale silk. 'Let's go shopping, unless you'd like some lunch first?'

After a leisurely lunch of pasta and salad, they went to Browns in South Molton Street, where Ali insisted Ursula had a short fitted dress, a short wool skirt, and two silk shirts. Ursula tried on a wide-brimmed black hat in Josephs, which made her green eyes appear mysterious and sultry, and admired a slinky cashmere jumper, but refused to buy them. 'Too extravagant Ali!' When they arrived at Selfridges in Oxford Street, she suddenly realised Ali was carrying them. 'My present to you Ursula, I insist!' As she picked up sensible leather shoes in Selfridges, Ali firmly took them from her grasp and put them back. Ursula reluctantly tried on elegant shoes in pale suede he waved at her. She stared mesmerised at her slender legs which unaccountably appeared much longer than she remembered. 'These shoes won't last long, Ali' she demurred. 'Oh for goodness' sake Ursula' he exclaimed, exasperated: 'You're not running the marathon in them. And you have to take that pair of slinky ankle boots too!' Later they bought a Dolce & Gabana beautifully cut, pale pink suit: 'That's it now Ali, and I will pay you back.' she said firmly. 'Okay' he said reluctantly. 'At least now, you'll look young and beautiful - the real you! Like a butterfly emerging from a dowdy old crysalis' he rhapsodised, hurriedly jumping away as she jokingly swung a carrier bag at him. But as they drove past Barkers in Kensington High Street he swung the Mercedes into a side street, miraculously finding a parking space. 'Come on' he pleaded, 'Just one more shop, let me buy you a present'
'Ali, you've already bought me two things.' she protested. 'What's money for, if not spending? I have plenty, and I want to spend it this way. You need a ski suit which I will get you tomorrow, as I want you to come ski-ing with me in December'

Ursula stared at him. 'And' he added hurriedly, 'now I will buy you another dress. The other one looks brilliant.'

Ursula and Ali were detained on the ground floor, by a persuasive sales assistant for a new non-cruelty cosmetics range. 'I don't mind if you want to try a make-over' said Ali, 'I can go and buy some shirts in the men's department.'
'Not a make-over' protested the woman as Ursula sat protected by a cape, with a light shining on her face. 'You're already pretty. Let's try out this light foundation, we can emphasise those high cheekbones with shader ...' Twenty minutes later Ursula looked at the result in the mirror, and was startled by the change. Her eyes looked enormous in her delicate face. 'I look like Twiggy in the sixties! A bit' she amended, worried that she sounded conceited. The shop assistant looked pleased: 'It's very fashionable at the moment'. On her way to meet Ali, Ursula tentatively tested Gautier's latest perfume. 'Have some more' said the assistant cheerfully, spraying it onto her wrist. Feeling she smelt too strongly of perfume and rather shy, Ursula found Ali in the men's department. He was laden with yet more carrier bags.

....

Actually Marius is beginning to get heavy, suffocating. I never thought I'd wish that he didn't like me so much. I don't feel guilty about taking his money for therapy, he shouldn't get it the way he does, but I don't like feeling under an obligation to him. The Sword of Damocles is poised above my head, I must get a proper job. Marius keeps ringing up now, even though he knows how I feel about 'phone calls. I don't like some of the guys he's begun hanging out with either, they're always off their heads. Last week I heard Malcolm making growling noises in the middle of the night. He was smashing open a cashbox with a hammer, down in the hall in the dark (someone has broken the light). No-one got up to investigate this time, not even Vivienne. That was the last time I stayed with Marius, he virtually begged me to. We didn't do anything. He's suddenly started showing an interest in Alex and asking questions about him, thank God he doesn't know about Gabriel.

****

Gabriel

At last I managed to speak to the girl who stands on the beer crate in Hammersmith Mall – yes! We met in Tesco's, of all romantic places, her name's Bubbles. Torquil began reminiscing about his conquests in supermarkets but I shut him up. I hope she doesn't think that I normally chat up the fairer sex in shops. I asked Bubbles where she applied all the gold paint and stuff and she said she did it in the loos at the Mall, that must be a drag. She lives miles away in Kentish Town, the Housing Co-op cheap set-up sounds great though. I gave her my number, I hope she rings me. We could go to *The Dove* for a drink, or perhaps she likes films? I could check what's on at Hammersmith Studios... Or meet half-way in town, go to the South Bank at Sunday lunchtime to hear music, she liked the busker. Oh please call me Bubbles, you're gorgeous. And you're not allergic to cats, I checked.

Big Girl is moored opposite us again. Torquil helped Matthew to sail her off to a berth on the visitors' pontoon before I went to the Edinburgh Festival. Torquil was thrilled, standing in the wheelhouse, steering the barge and looking like something from a 1950's *Boys Annual*. The boat only collided with the pier because the propeller fell off. No harm was done and Torquil has begun subscribing to the RBOA and nagging me about him living in the hold permanently. I need my space, rent or no rent; anyway I don't want the boat rocking when he uses it as a gay knocking shop. To be honest, part of the reason Torquil is here, is because I need to be needed. I should stop this tendency as apparently it can be akin to a disease, in which case I'm terminally ill.

Matthew is back because he didn't want to lose his berth to two enormous boats that appeared at the pontoon last week. Apparently the *Clashing Rooms* TV crew were performing a transformation of a room on each boat. Judging by past efforts (I've watched it occasionally on Stuart's television) it'll be a couple of theatre sets based on MDF, bonding agents, emulsion, Sophia's sprayed-on jeans, plus a lot of effort. For a couple of heady days a strong smell of glue permeated the air as far as St. Nicholas' graveyard, while the *Pissed Up!* bar on the bank rocked. Then the TV transits departed, and the din of ducks fighting could be heard once more. Torquil was his usual embarrassing self. As a man who never recognises celebrities, when he saw Quentin Lewd-Bollard on the quay, Torquil thought he knew him from a Club and gaily pinched his bottom. Old Bollard nearly fell in the river. Torquil's definitely not moving onto the boat now, too un-cool.

Another reason he isn't is because I'm a bit tired of people assuming I'm gay. I have no objection *per se* but the word's spreading, and I would like another heterosexual relationship some time before I'm 35. Ironically I've spotted Paula, Matthew's 15-year-old daughter, looking longingly at Torquil from the wheelhouse of *Big Girl*. Torquil is one of those annoyingly beautiful people who look as though they've just left a photoshoot for 'Vogue', when they've been out carousing all night. She's probably seen him bringing me morning coffee, clad decoratively in his Dims. He then flits around dusting, while I slump on the sofa depressing myself with yesterday's newspaper before scrambling out to work. I looked up today in time to see the postman - whom Torquil yearns after – staring through the window at this scene of domestic bliss. Good job I'd remembered to don my sarong.

Torquil and I met the owner of one of the boats transformed by *Clashing Rooms*, at the pub.
'What's it like?' I asked. The guy was pale. 'Awful,' he said, 'I'm Chris by the way' he added, a bit nonplussed, as Torquil beamed lustfully at him. He's about to sail back to Chelsea where he's usually moored in the middle of the river, with no amenities. This apparently costs him over £2000 a year, perhaps Chiswick Pier isn't as over-priced as I thought it was. Torquil now assumes Chris is rich.
'What do you do about about sewage?' asked Torquil, trying to sound knowledgeable by apeing the type of intellectual conversation boat people have.
'Into the Thames,' said the millionaire, sucking a boiled sweet with gusto.
I go swimming in that.

'It washes all round *The Ark*,' Torquil said gleefully, flicking a glance at me. That's the last time he uses my bathroom to wax his trunk line while I'm clearing rubbish from the water outside.

Please ring me Bubbles, you've got four years before I'm 35, but I'd really like to hear from you now.

****

Bubbles

I was talking to Rosalie in the kitchen today and she seemed sweet, if rather boring. I caught her looking at me with faint incredulity once or twice, particularly when I did my anti-capitalist rant. She's been staying in the back room for a few weeks now, but I scarcely ever see her as she found herself a Temp day job and a waitressing evening job soon after she arrived. I was a bit intimidated by her at the Co-Op meeting when she did the Minutes, but actually I think she's shy. It transpired that she was throwing out all these wonderful clothes she'd bought and didn't like, I couldn't believe my luck when she asked if I wanted them. The clothes are not the sort I'd usually buy, as they're rather conventional and definitely expensive. Luckily they're not Matilda's thing at all: she doesn't need many clothes with her job. Being serious for a moment, she prefers living in jeans and raids charity shops for exotic bits for her stage act. Rosalie's clothes look surprisingly good on me. I'm going to have my hair trimmed too. I can't wait to wow Alex ... And it'll be good practice for meeting Gabriel.

****

Romance

Ascending the escalators inside the tasteful tranquility of the department store, Ursula felt young and excited. She had been cautious for so long, that now she could hardly absorb the huge changes that she had set in motion. Well, not totally her, she thought, the catalyst had been Anthony. Ali saw the smile leave her face and the sadness in her long-lashed eyes.

'Hey' he said, nudging her gently, 'what's up?' 'Oh, nothing' said Ursula brightly, walking off the escalator quickly into the women's clothing department.

She could hear Ali charming the sales woman as she hurriedly changed again, this time into a white mini-dress that left her arms bare. The low scooped neck and back showed off her arms and shoulders: she tried to pull it higher over her cleavage. Her fingers fumbled with the buckle of the belt which emphasised her slim waist. 'Goodness!' thought Ursula, craning over her shoulder. She carefully put on her new shoes. Thank goodness she still had a faint tan from the summer.
'Come on Ursula, let's see' Ali called.

She shyly emerged. Ali and the sales woman beamed at her 'I'm buying that for you, no protests!' said Ali, spinning her round by the shoulder to face the mirror. Ursula pulled her heavy hair over one shoulder so that it swung down over one breast. She stared at the vision that faced her, breathlessly. She looked young, alluring and beautiful. Tears suddenly filled her eyes 'Oh Ali, thank you!' she said impetuously kissing him on the cheek.

'Ursula, is that you?' the familiar voice sounded very uncertain. With amazement, Ursula turned and saw Sarah hurrying across the shop between the rails of clothing. 'Ursula, you look marvellous' she breathed. 'Oh' she saw Ali, and her eyes quickly took in the ring glittering on Ursula's wedding finger. 'Oh Ursula, congratulations! I didn't know you'd got married.'
'It was a very quiet wedding' said Ursula hurriedly, hearing a note of hurt in Sarah's voice. 'This is Ali, Ali this is my friend Sarah.'
'Hello Sarah' said Ali warmly, shaking her hand.
'I'm sorry I haven't been in touch Sarah, I've ...been busy'
'Obviously' said Sarah with a world of understatement.
'Seriously though, I'm really happy for you both. I never realised that that was why you moved- Oh, there's Anthony. Anthony!' she called 'over here'.

Ursula froze and for a second all sounds stopped; she thought she might faint then pulled herself together. She turned slowly and saw Anthony walking towards her. His eyes travelled over her incredulously. Did she imagine the spark of admiration? 'Doesn't Ursula look wonderful?' asked Sarah, 'and this is Ali, her new husband'.

'We've met' said Anthony, coldly nodding at Ali, who was looking unusually bland. Ursula stared at them both, curiosity overcoming her embarrassment. Anthony looked back at her, she blushed and restrained the impulse to pull her hem down and neckline up. 'Congratulations' he said formally. 'Come on Sarah, or I'll be late. Good-bye'. Sarah grimaced after the tall departing figure, with a what's-the-matter-with-him look: 'Ring me Ursula' she said, kissing her on the cheek . 'Yes of course' said Ursula warmly, feeling contemptible for having avoided her old friend.

'I didn't know you knew him' said Ali resentfully as they reached the flat, after a subdued drive home. 'He's the man I had the disagreement with at 'Clouds', he owns it, and he's my old landlord', explained Ursula reluctantly. She followed Ali into the lift. She was still trying to recover her poise; it was terrifying that someone could affect her so much.

'I didn't realise it was him,' said Ali, 'Mind you, it fits. He always acts as if he's God' he added venomously. Ursula didn't recognise this vindictive side of Ali. 'Why don't you like him?' she asked.

'He poached one of my best jockeys two years ago, plus I'm sure it was him who tipped off the authorities when-' Ali stopped abruptly. Ursula looked at him in consternation; how many illegal things was Ali involved in? 'It's okay sweet Ursula' he joked, his face hidden as he let her precede him into the flat, 'you're the only illegal thing in my life.' Ursula felt uneasily she didn't believe this, but Ali's good humour was restored. 'Promise.' he said, smiling at her anxious face while he filled the kettle. He spooned coffee into the cafetiere whistling quietly.

Ursula had noticed that if the phone rang for Ali, he would run upstairs to take the call in his office with the door closed. She rather wondered why she hadn't met any of his friends yet - but then he hadn't met hers, she excused. Apart from Sarah

of course. Their lives had fallen into their separate routines. Ali was out all night at least once a week, leaving home in the late evening looking very spruce and returning at breakfast time, pale and unshaven. One evening she saw him putting a thick wad of £50 banknotes in his pocket, and wondered where he went. Fatima expressed ignorance when Ursula mentioned it.
'Maybe he goes out to gamble, playing cards?'

Bracing herself, Ursula rang Jane and Paula and arranged to meet them one evening at a Chinese Restaurant, near Leicester Square. 'I've got some surprising news for you' she promised. She could feel they were intrigued, but only laughed when Jane asked if she was going on holiday. The best Paula could manage was to ask whether Ursula had found another job. There was no mention of men, she noticed with some chagrin. It had obviously never crossed her friends' minds that she could be sexually attractive. It would be a relief though to tell them she was married - it seemed to make it more legal rather than less, for some reason. She hadn't told her family, only phoning them to say she had moved in order *to share a better flat with a friend.*

....

'Hold on Marius, I'm not sure whether she's back yet.' Chloris put her hand over the 'phone receiver in the sitting-room and looked round enquiringly at Bubbles. Bubbles shook her head violently, her face rigid with tension and tiptoed back into the kitchen where she was making toast. 'No she's not here... Yes, I did tell her you called yesterday. Yes, I will tell her....Bye.'

Bubbles remembered causing Marius to smile, stutter, and lose the thread of conversation by glancing at him across a crowded room. This after only one eventful Sunday afternoon spent, in all senses, in his room. They had had only to glance flirtatiously at one another to relive their passion in full technicolour. The power trip was addictive. He'd smelt of bonfires, she should have been warned.

What had changed? She'd met Alex, and now Gabriel.
Bubbles had been unable to borrow Matilda's mobile as she
was away visiting friends, so she had steeled herself and
visited the 'phone box at the end of the road. She'd
breathlessly left a message with Gabriel's housemate that
she'd called, but in the stress of the moment she couldn't
remember her home 'phone number, so had quickly rung off.

****

Therapy Session

Alex emerged hurriedly onto the pavement from the staircase
down to the basement room, closing the iron gate behind him.
I'd been standing lost on the wide wet pavement in the
twilight, wondering where he was after ringing the door-bell
fruitlessly outside the consulting-room.
'I'm sorry about this Undine, because it's late, someone's
booked the other room. We'll go to my flat as there are still
papers everywhere in the basement.'
I was surprised that he remembered my name, I didn't always
think he did during earlier sessions.
'A peripatetic existence,' I observed as we hurried back along
the street beneath the cold lights and warm drizzle.
'No,' he said sharply, 'Those days are gone, thank goodness.'

'This is a change of style,' Ax said, looking appreciatively over
his shoulder at me as he unlocked the front door. I was glad
he preceded me up the communal carpeted stairs, as my skirt
was uncharacteristically short, and new dainty sandals *a la
mode Rosalie* caused me to wobble slightly on unaccustomed
heels. The light ticked away on a time switch in the hall as I
waited for him to open the door to the apartment. I was
aware of a large shadowed sitting-room yawning on my left as
I followed him along the hall. There was sisal carpeting on
the floor of the narrow dining-room. It smelt evocatively of the
squat Helena and I had made habitable in Islington. Oil
paintings were stacked against the wall, a French clock ticked
lightly. Lighting from three shaded wall lamps illuminated the
high full bookcase behind him and gave him an artificial halo.
'I met a woman at a support group I went to in Tufnell Park,
on Thursday,' I said proudly.

Ax nodded abstractedly, laying out his files neatly on the dining-table.

'She hasn't got OCD any more – it's vanished. I'll be cured too.'

'I don't use the 'c' word,' he said quickly.

I laughed. Cunt. I was tempted to say it, nothing wrong with a bit of good old Anglo-Saxon. I became aware that I wasn't worried about touching the lacquered table.

'You should read this book,' I advised enthusiastically. 'I think you'd enjoy it, it's really good.'

'I don't read fiction as a rule, but let's have a look.' I almost mentioned Georgette Heyer, but decided not to.

He turned the paperback over and looked at the photograph of Richard Ford on the cover.

'Maybe I will.'

'Another good one is –'

'I think we need to carry on, Undine.'

I handed over the Anxiety Log, suddenly nervous. 'Sorry, I didn't manage to do it on Sunday.'

	Mon.	Tues.	Wed.	Thurs.	Fri	Sat.	Sun.
Taps	4	8	6	7	7	8	
Iron	5	7	8	7	6	5	
Stove	6	6	6	7	6	6	
Doors	4	5	6	5	4	6	

'Do you remember what happened where the scores rise again here, what triggered off the anxiety?'

I tried to remember. 'I think I was late for work, which makes the OCD worse. And I was tired.'

Sleep is still problematic, particularly if I start worrying about getting enough of it. I studied the book case behind him.

'For someone who doesn't read fiction, there's quite a bit on those shelves.'

Alex leaned back in his chair, smiling at me for the first time, then twisted away to look down and pulled a tatty paperback from a low shelf.

'You read poems,' I exclaimed approvingly.

'Yes, this is one of my favourites. It's a bit naughty.'

I felt myself shrink back imperceptibly, then he was saying in beautifully modulated tones:

'To His Coy Mistress'

Alex gave me a wicked sideways glance, then read on:

Had we but world enough, and time,
This coyness, lady, were no crime.
We would sit down, and think which way
To walk, and pass our long love's day.
Thou by the Indian Ganges' side
Shoudst rubies find; I by the tide
Of Humber would complain. I would
Love you ten years before the flood,
And you should, if you please, refuse
Till the conversion of the Jews.
My vegetable love should grow
Vaster than empires and more slow;
An hundred years should go to praise
Thine eyes, and on thy forehead gaze;
Two hundred to adore each breast,
But thirty thousand to the rest;
An age at least to every part,
And the last age should show your heart.
For, lady, you deserve this state,
Nor would I love at lower rate.
But at my back I always hear
Time's wingéd chariot hurrying near;
And yonder all before us lie
Deserts of vast eternity.
Thy beauty shall no more be found;
Nor, in thy marble vault, shall sound
My echoing song; then worms shall try
That long-preserved virginity,
And your quaint honor turn to dust,
And into ashes all my lust:
The grave's a fine and private place,
But none, I think, do there embrace.
Now therefore, while the youthful hue
Sits on thy skin like morning dew,
And while thy willing soul transpires
At every pore with instant fires,
Now let us sport us while we may,

And now, like amorous birds of prey,
Rather at once our time devour
Than languish in his slow-chapped power.
Let us roll all our strength and all
Our sweetness up into one ball,
And tear our pleasures with rough strife
Thorough the iron gates of life:
Thus, though we cannot make our sun
Stand still, yet we will make him run.

I couldn't look at Ax. I stared at the un-curtained leaded window.
'That was beautiful.' He'd obviously forgotten that I'd included an excerpt from the poem by Andrew Marvell in my novel. But I would have yielded if I'd been the coy mistress: Ax is not to know that reading romantic literature in a sexy voice to me constitutes foreplay. Or perhaps he'd guessed. I crossed my legs, then remembered the short skirt and hurriedly uncrossed them, placing my knees primly together
'You can borrow the book if you like,' Ax offered reluctantly.
'But you'd have to remember to let me have it back.'
'Oh no, thanks, I don't want to. I can't touch borrowed things without worrying yet.'
His eyes sharpened with interest, seeing a challenge. He looked like a satyr in the reddish light. I remarked upon the flamboyant, loving, handwriting on the flyleaf: 'Oh, some old dear gave it to me,' he said dismissively, replacing the book on the shelf.

'Time to finish.'
I rose without touching the table or chair. Suddenly Ax hurried to the heavy door, opened it and before I could reluctantly take the handle, it had slammed behind him. I stood stranded on my heels, anxiety level seven. He reappeared after long minutes, 'I thought you were behind me.'
'You vanished.'
'Just making sure the coast is clear, I don't want you running into any family members. I wouldn't do that to you.'
You're lying, you're embarrassed by me. One of your Nutters.

I wonder what his wife and daughter are like? Is his wife brunette, Jewish, blond, Negroid, intelligent or sensible? Is he the more sensitive and highly-strung partner? Or is she glamorous, dizzy and wealthy? Did he sneer when I mentioned that I work hard renovating the places in which I live? But physical labour was my philosophy, and a way in which I challenged gender and class stereotyping, and my fastidiousness. This year though, I've stopped lifting and carrying very heavy things, it's supposed to be bad for women. I would like to have a child after all. It's probably too late, I'm too damaged.

****

Gabriel

Torquil went walking in the Alps at 5:30 this morning. He thundered off the boat being laboriously quiet. 'The Sound of Music' intermingled with Sounds of Torquil trickled through duvet pulled over my head, he'd left the CD playing softly. The cats promptly decamped onto my back and legs, purring loudly and scratching. The flea collars were obviously not working again and Gin was trying to eat his. I capitulated and lurched into the sitting-room, yawning. Stuck to the 'fridge was a note from Torquil wishing me a good week. I resignedly switched on 'Farming Today' and blearily prepared a full cafetiere of coffee to jump-start a new day at the hospital.

Abigail is determined to nest on *The Ark* (even the sloping roof at one point, judging by the thuds from overhead) with four cats sitting open-jawed below, waiting for toppling fluffy ducklings. Not known for their brains, ducks. Her quest for a nest leads to constant furious quacking at dawn, and cat fights for the best ringside seat. I'm so exhausted that I've answered the phone 'MFI Unit' at work a couple of times. Despite this the hospital still seems to value my services. The cats haven't tackled Aggressive Abigail, but if Tonic absent-mindedly sits on her one of these days, she'll be two-dimensional.

The groups of school kids on the river bank comment pungently on the distinctive smell of the mud at low tide and, as I hang my jeans over the railings outside to dry, Florence has promised to tell me if I smell of Thames mud. At least there's no longer any risk of me smelling of baked beans from washing up in the bath: the new kitchen sink is *in situ* which has improved the quality of life aboard considerably.

....

I haven't heard from Bubbles, I keep checking my mobile.

Yesterday the trees on the opposite bank appeared romantically misty – nothing to do with early summer light, it was through a pall of smoke from Mark setting fire to the hold. Initially, he was harmlessly chain-sawing planks out of the ceiling. Dan from next door told me he could hear the work punctuated by surprised exclamations of 'Ouch!' and 'They're falling on me 'ead!' Mark then apparently sawed industriously at a metal bolt until it was white hot and sparks fell into wood shavings he'd left on the floor below. These smouldered happily, miraculously not bursting into flame, while he was off having acupuncture. I hope he said 'Ouch!' there too. I'm so relieved Torquil is still on holiday, he'd have freaked – plus about the black oily finger and boot prints Mark leaves all over the upper deck.

Apparently everyone on the pontoon thought I knew that Mark, although trading as an electrician, can't get insurance nowadays to carry so much as a matchbox. Trust me to hire Pyromaniac & Son. When I told Mark that I'd been frightened arriving home from work to see smoke seeping out through the closed portholes, and pointed out that I would be homeless without the uninsured Ark, he said, 'Oh don't Gabe, you'll frighten me!'. He laughed uproariously. He went on to decry the reek of smoke, saying it would have been better if there had been flames as then there wouldn't be this horrible smell. When Mark lit some incense sticks I sacked him, but he cunningly misunderstood and said kindly that he didn't like breaking off jobs in the middle. When I had a vivid vision of drowning him ('Ouch, the water's cold!') I left for work early to avoid temptation.

It didn't save me: Mark jauntily strolled into the hospital Reception Area this afternoon. Apparently he lives nearby - probably c/o HM prison across the road, judging by the dodgy junction box he's installed on the boat.

'I could tell you some stories from my other jobs, Gabe,' he said rashly, breathing halitosis across the desk and winking unwisely at Florence. I hate people abbreviating my name. Mark said he'd just dropped by to mention that he wasn't sure if he had locked up at the boat: 'and there are loads of kids messing about on the pontoon'. When I asked him to go back and check, he came back with a rambling excuse, digressing fit for a stage act. Fortunately the patient behind him in the queue elbowed him aside, before he became one.

Maisie likened Mark to Homer Simpson when I told her in a quiet moment that Mark had pulled out two of Torquil's toy trolls from the back of the bathroom cupboard, and placed them on the shelf kissing romantically. I cycled home from work today like a bat out of hell - Nemesis seems to be moonlighting as Mark – to find the front door double-locked.

After spending some of the Bank Holiday trying to clean indelible evidence of Mark's Doc Martens from the hall carpet and washing brown oily stains from the washing machine (bit of a mystery that), microwave, doors, walls and the exterior of Torquil's white kettle for the fourth day running, I left a polite note asking Mark to remove his shoes indoors and giving permission for kettle to be used in the hold. Torquil's due back in a couple of days' time and I don't need more hassle. The kettle now remains in situ in the sitting room, reproachfully pristine, but as herbal tea and coffee is disappearing fast my conscience is clear. I'm sure Mark's wiped his feet on Torquil's lilac bath towel though, nobody's hands are that big. I keep my towel separately in the bedroom now, hanging over the four-poster. It's not that I'm fussy, in fact girlfriends used to accuse me of being scruffy, but Mark is medieval in his horror of water. He was about to change out of his work clothes in front of me in the sitting room one evening, without washing, and I banished him to the hall. I could hear him spraying himself liberally with deodorant, over the top of his 'bird-pulling gear'. As he left, springing heavily down onto the pontoon, a feral scent of Calvin Klein with woody bass tones of soot and sweat trailed behind him.

****

Romance

Ursula was slow to realise she now had a whole new look, a different existence - in fact it was beginning to feel like a new personae. She didn't always recognise the sophisticated young woman who looked flirtatiously back at her from the long mirror in her room. The new facets of her personality hadn't emerged from her marriage though, Ursula realised with a sudden shock, they were what had led to it. Attributable to Anthony again - meeting him was when she first began behaving out of character. She could not put blame on him thought, the decision to marry had been hers. But he had put her in a very difficult position, another part of her mind objected. Giving up the problem, Ursula threw her hairbrush down crossly. Why did he have such an impact on her? In his mind, she thought miserably, she probably ranked in importance somewhere below a nylon cardigan. One result of the encounter in Barkers, was that Ursula was forced to acknowledge she could never settle down with Ali. The way the room had spun at a glance from Anthony's slate-blue eyes, and images of his lean powerful frame haunted her thoughts. He was the most masculine man she had ever met, she thought, momentarily overwhelmed.

'You weren't joking!' shrieked Paula, briefly silencing the chatter at tables around them. 'I hardly recognised you Ursula, that dress is gorgeous and the hat...And I kept telling you to wear your hair down, didn't I?' she asked smugly. 'I haven't told you the news yet' said Ursula laughing despite herself at Paula's excitement, and Jane's stunned expression. Four men seated at the next table stared at her admiringly as she sat down. Ursula looked at her friends then placed her left hand on the table, the diamonds flashed. Jane's eyes widened. 'You're married! Oh, wow. How wonderful! Who to?' she asked breathlessly. Both friends' questions and exclamations

took up much of the main course of assorted Chinese dishes. Jane however sensed something amiss: 'Ursula, are you okay? You seem, well, a bit quiet?'

'Oh yes,' Ursula hastened to reassure her. 'Everything's fine. I'm probably just a bit shell-shocked too.'

'It's all been very fast' said Paula bluntly. 'If it was anyone but you Ursula, I'd be wondering about shotgun weddings' she giggled. 'Or marriages of convenience!' Ursula almost choked and reached blindly for her glass of water. Oblivious, Paula related the tale of a friend who had entered such an arrangement. 'He was horrible' Paula said with relish. 'Just wanted to stay here to keep up his shady connections. The police came and arrested him in the end.' Blushing, Ursula hoped fervently that Paula wasn't predicting Ali's future. Paula prattled on: 'She was supposed to stay with him three years-'

'Sorry?' said Ursula sharply. She felt her skin prickle with dismay. Three years, Ali had only said one. Paula and Jane stared at her: 'I didn't know it was that long.' Ursula tried to speak calmly.

'Anyway, you haven't married for convenience, not with that ring' said Jane stolidly, to Ursula's relief. 'We want to meet him'.

'Yes, you must come over soon' said Ursula. She spent the rest of the evening both dreading and longing to confront Ali.

'I didn't know it was three years' Ali said avoiding her accusing look as she stood in front of him.

'Ali, you must have done! How could you and Fatima have deceived me like that? I thought you were my friends.' Ursula paced the sitting room, distressed and angry. She also silently blamed herself: what an idiot! Fancy trusting Ali and Fatima, and not finding out more for herself. She looked across at him seated in the armchair, head bent.

'Well I hoped.. I hoped you'd change your mind Ursula. You know, enjoyed living with me enough to-' Ali broke off.

'Become your proper wife you mean? But I made it really clear that that wouldn't happen, Ali.'

'Yes' he admitted. He was now fiddling miserably with the dvd remote.

Despite herself Ursula felt a wave of pity for him; 'I shouldn't have put such a strain on you, I knew you...loved me. Oh Ali.'

'What are you going to do?' he looked up pleadingly, his face pale.

'My promise to stay a year doesn't mean anything now. I can't stay here now Ali, not if we are to have any sort of friendship left in future.' Ursula said more gently. I've been looking for a job, and when I get one, I'll move out.'

Ursula pulled off the ring and laid it on the table. Ali didn't say anything. She went to her room and stared unseeingly out of the window at the illuminated outline of Harrods and the rows of car headlights. The scene blurred with angry tears. When she turned she saw a new white Nevika ski suit laid out on her bed.

There was a light tap at the door; Ali stood awkwardly in the corridor.

'Ursula, please, please come skiing with me, you can move out after that.'

'No, Ali' she said blinking back her tears.'

'Please, we both need a holiday, and anyway I've booked it all - to go to Les Arcs in France. I can't cancel without losing a lot of money.'

She wavered.

'Go on, then you can move out when you want to. I won't put any pressure on you, honestly.'

'Maybe' she said hesitantly. His face brightened with relief, 'But Ali, there is no chance of me changing my mind about us, about anything.'

'Fine, fine' he said hurriedly.

'All right then' she agreed slowly. Ursula heard Ali humming later, as though he hadn't believed her. 'Hope springs eternal' she thought, then realised sadly that applied to her too, but about someone else.

Her absolute priority now was to get a job, Ursula thought. She would pay Ali back for the new clothes he'd bought her, and leave. She rang Sarah at work; a young unknown voice answered. '.And who shall I say is calling?' Ursula told her and waited.

'Hi Ursula, how's married life?' asked Sarah with wonderful timing. There was silence.

'Ursula, are you still there?'

'Yes. Umm Sarah, I'm looking for another job so if you hear of anything...' Ursula's voice shook. Sarah realised all wasn't well, but with monumental tact didn't probe.

'I'm really sorry Ursula' she said regretfully, 'But I had to take someone on when you said you weren't coming back.'

'Of course you did' said Ursula warmly. She couldn't have borne working at 'Clouds' again anyway, with the ever-present risk of running into Anthony.

Ursula gave Naomi Sarah's glowing reference, and they discussed the vacancy over coffee. The pay was very good; there seemed a lot of potential in the shop which was effectively the new manageress's to manage and buy for as she wished. 'A young woman called Sophie works here too, as an assistant.' said Naomi fixing Ursula with piercing blue eyes. 'She's at the dentist this morning. Sophie's only 19, but very responsible and easy to get on with. She's been here for about six months. I'm afraid I have two other people to see, so I'll try to let you know what I decide by Monday. You have an excellent CV though.'

They said good-bye, and Ursula walked along towards Piccadilly Circus occasionally smiling up at the bright blue sky. Her heart lifted optimistically. Life seemed to be looking up.

Ursula went to visit her parents for the day at their terraced house in Ruislip. They seemed pleased to see her, but as usual, totally preoccupied with their own world.

'You do look smart dear,' her mother said approvingly. 'Have you had your hair done? I thought of having mine done. When I was in Windsor with Daphne the other day, we saw this new hairdressers and I said...' For the next twenty minutes, Ursula listened patiently, making appropriate noises whenever her mother stopped to draw breath.

Her father said vaguely over lunch of cold meat and vegetables, 'You've moved then?'

Her mother broke off from a monologue about the neighbour's dogs. 'Is your new flatmate nice? We'll come up and see you when I feel stronger.'

'Well,' Ursula said hesitantly, girding herself to lie about Ali, but she needn't have worried. Her mother didn't wait for an *answer before launching into a familiar lament. This referred self-pityingly to the fact that Ursula had the freedom to have a good time, that she could only have dreamt of when she was young. For the first time, instead of misery at her mother's difficult life, Ursula felt a deep reviving anger at both parents' selfishness. This helped her to leave them early, and without her usual anxiety about them.*

****

Gabriel

It's 7.20am! Mark is standing inside my sitting room blocking the exit and haranguing me about needing £500 more than he quoted. I can see why Torquil is so keen on locking the front door at night now. I said I couldn't afford to pay more and reminded Mark to screw down the new floorboards downstairs, not nail them, as I needed to be able to lift them to check for leaks. He suddenly became so vague he shimmered, but it might just have been the smell of varnish. I think Mark was hoping to hide all the mounds of rubbish in the hold under the floor, rather than take the sacks of soot, a chemical lavatory and rusty anchor chains to the dump in his van as promised. He said defiantly: 'I ain't got no roof rack.'
'Which means you have. Oh never mind, I thought you had.'
'It fell off, Thursday, lucky there was nothing behind me.'
'But it's a large Transit...'
'It's full though.'
I had to ask. 'What with?'
'Things I might need.'
Sounds like Sheila's handbag syndrome to me. I reluctantly left for work, leaving Mark sitting on the bench on the deck admiring the view, pondering his huge workload and blowing on his tea. I didn't mention the kissing trolls. I'll make sure the front door's locked tomorrow morning, then if Mark hurls himself at it he'll bounce off into the Thames.

I wish Bubbles would get in touch. Maybe I'll do some shopping in Hammersmith Mall on the way home, it's been six days.

The vast slab of beech to be sawn up for the kitchen worktop has been delivered two weeks early – naturally, as we don't need it yet. I helped the Geordie chap, who was plump and hard-faced, to carry it down the ramp to the boat. Heavy deliveries always happen at low tide when the ramp has a 1-in-2 slope, so we ended up hurtling headlong towards the water with little dancing steps. The slab is laid flat on the sitting room floor as it can't be stored on its side. It weighs a ton or whatever the metric equivalent is, and takes up the whole room.

Torquil's back, and making cross noises every time he trips over the edge of the beech. At the moment he's lying on the sofa reading magazines, surrounded by enchanted cats, exhausted by having shown me a miniscule blister on his heel caused by his pristine walking boots. He's sorted out Mark though, which is a relief (we're now paying him only £150 extra). I'm even glad to hear Torquil's familiar snorting. Torquil always sniffs journals and books before reading them. He says the cool, water-smooth, glue-scented pages of magazines in particular are fantastic for the senses. It does dull the enjoyment, him having buried his beak lasciviously in Lance Armstrong's crotch, when I just want to enjoy my new copy of *Cycling Monthly*.

****

Bubbles

Matilda's back today so I'll be able to text Gabriel, I don't know what to say. I've been off work this week with 'flu. I keep trying out different messages: writing them down, saying them aloud. I'm really excited, but also deadly scared. Maybe the work with Ax will help me to have a calm relationship with Gabriel, I doubt it though. Anyway I still lust after Ax almost all the time, although I don't like him as much as I did. Dislike has always lent an erotic edge though, take Marius. Part of being overwhelmed by Ax could be because he knows about OCD, unlike anyone I've met before. It gives him a lot of power. It's weird to think that we grew up almost part of the same generation and he's made his work a study of my mental condition.

I want to see Alex's notes about me; be funny if they're shopping lists. Perhaps he'll be up until eleven o'clock one night grumpily making up OCD symptoms for me to read.

****

Therapy Session

'How did you get on with the Anxiety Log?' Ax asked, busily sorting out papers, 'Have a seat.'
'I didn't do it.'
'Why not?' He sounded normal and was still looking down, but I suddenly felt anger emanating from him.
'Well… I wasn't quite sure how to do it, and … I rebelled.'
'Acceptance would be a good thing to think about Undine,' he said quietly, sitting opposite me in the chair. He wrote something on the sheet.
'What did you write?' I demanded, suddenly fearful.
Alex raised his hands in mock surrender. 'Just "not sure how to do Anxiety Log"', he said.
I can't tell you what I did to my brother, because you write things down and I wouldn't want you ever to record that or anything connected with it.
Ax was sitting back, surveying me, idly undoing the buttons on his red shirt cuffs and folding the sleeves back.
Daringly I said: 'I would like to be able to see my notes because it worries me, when you write things down.'
'Yes, of course you can. You may not be able to understand my scrawl though.'
'You write neatly.' His arms are muscular.
'I mean, my shorthand.'
'Thanks for saying I can see them, it just worries me. Things seem to be going so slowly. Is there, well, is there cause for concern?'
'Things aren't going that slowly, you're writing and we've done some exposure work,' he sounded defensive.
'How would I know if you thought I needed to go to hospital?'

'How do you think?'

'I don't know. I hope, that you'd ask me first or warn me?'

'I would talk it over with you, and maybe someone close to you and recommend that you see one of my colleagues.'*

Silence, while I try and trust him.

'We can't get any further without me telling you what I did to my brother can we?'

His beautiful eyes concentrated on me and he smiled slightly in assent and leaned forward.

'Why don't you?'

'Because I think it would cause more problems than it solved.' I said carefully.

'It comes down to a lack of trust, that's interesting.' That sounded like the standard glib response when therapists can't think of anything else to say.

'I think it was because you were hard to get hold of during the first few weeks.'

'I'll buy that.'

'If I told you Alex, whenever you said anything afterwards, I would be wondering whether you were referring to what I'd told you, or passing judgement. I'd jump on your every word.'

When we both lean forward like this, it would be so easy to kiss him.

'What happens if people tell you something that they can be arrested for?'

'Undine, this is important. I would tell the Police or authorities if a child is, present tense, in danger, or if I felt that I was at risk. Only in those circumstances.'

I leaned back, I still couldn't tell him.

'Do you think that you would shock me?' he asked with an edge of incredulity.

Others have been shocked, why not you Sunshine? Anyway, I'm tempted to do something bad now, just to shock you out of that complacency.

....

That night Bubbles had a vivid dream about Ax; she did not usually take account of her dreams. She realised after a while during a session that Ax was drunk; he was not responding to her signals of speech and eye contact. It was reminiscent of trying to talk to Grania when she was a child, except that Grania hadn't been inebriated, just in her own distant, hostile world. After a short time Ax began smoking openly, he offered her a cigarette. She knew this behaviour to be unusual, usually Ax tried to conceal the fact he was a smoker. She thought she ought to make a note on a medical form, open a file for him. She looked for a blue file to differentiate him from other patients. She became aware that there were children, his, sitting in a row on the sofa of the sitting-room. It was a low white-washed basement room, very similar to the kitchen of Marius's house. A couple of women were quietly moving around the kitchen and staircase nearby, leading their own lives.

As he bent towards her Ax's skin appeared coarsened in the lamplight, his hair shaggy. He moved closer, he smelt of smoke and whisky. She became aware that a shift had occurred, with difficulty she realised that she had to look after him.

'Come on, let's get you a cab,' she said. She'd heard other people saying efficient things like that, but they had money.

****

Gabriel

I saw Bubbles! She was strolling into Hammersmith tube station in a pink dress, she looked very pretty and her hair is different. I couldn't get through the crowds quickly enough before she was through the barrier and had rounded the corner into the passage. I shouted her name and would have vaulted the barrier as there were queues for tickets, but it was the rush-hour and the turnstiles were congested with a tidal wave of robotic, blankly-staring commuters marching towards me.

I've just got home and found a text message from her. I left my mobile behind this morning. She says she can meet up a week on Wednesday – I'm so happy. When I 'phone the mobile to agree to this plan, an impersonal message service picks up.

The cats are draped langorously all over the only comfortable sofa, it used to be white, expressionlessly watch me playing air guitar and dancing around enthusiastically to the Arctic Monkeys. All this while ironing shirts for work – who says men can't multi-task?

****

Therapy Session

Perhaps I should stop going to see Ax; it's getting worse again since he read me the poem. He's my first thought as I wake, and last image in my mind as I fall asleep, hand between my legs. If I tell him how I feel, will he look affronted, pleased, smug, loving, frightened, embarrassed, disgusted? I dress with great care for our sessions, choosing clothes a week in advance. I diet, shower and wax and scent and oil my body, and carefully apply cosmetics to my smooth face. Alone, I sing to him, talk to him, dream about him, exercise for him, think about him, hear his voice, hope for him, fantasise about him … How I fantasise about him! I couldn't bear it if he looked horrified or complacent. I can't tell the man how devastatingly attractive I find him. Ax has said that I'm interesting. I've just realised: being informed that you are interesting by a Psychotherapist is not necessarily a compliment. I should stop going to see him. I can't.

****

Gabriel

My closest link to meditation is to close my eyes and visualise the pure lines and clean elegance of an empty ordinary large brown cardboard box. Then I-
'You're obviously destined to live on the streets then, aren't you Torq?'
'Gabriel, don't creep up on me!'
'Sorry. Is that all you've written?'
'The creative process can't be rushed.'
'I thought you loved being a freelance designer.'
'Oh I do, but I'm so creative it just sort of rushes out in all directions. What's so funny?'

'Well don't give up the day job.'
'Thanks.'
'Don't mention it, I came to ask if you want me to turn down your asparagus soup.'
'Ooh, look!' Torquil hooted maliciously as 'Sperm over the Internet' flashed up as a News item at the bottom of the screen. 'Tell that to Sheila, the broody mare, she could sit astride her Pentium 3!'
Gabriel flinched at the graphic image. Thank goodness he'd got Broadband, Torquil used the Net more often than a fisherman.
'Are you still in touch with her?' he asked nervously.
'Yes, Sheila's all right - but then again she's not after my body.'
'Burning asparagus anyone?'
While Torquil was in the kitchen, Gabriel tried to look at his Bank account on-line but discovered he'd forgotten his 'Memorable Information' password.

****

Bubbles

Here I am again, walking along the wide hall ahead of him, left into the drawing-room. Something seems different, I can't quite put my finger on it. Ax is looking pleasantly bland. As usual, we take our accustomed positions. 'You look as though you might run away,' he says, indicating my ubiquitous plastic carrier bag between my ankles as I perch on the edge of my seat.
'I'm frightened things will fall out.'
'Ah,' he writes something quickly on the sheet of paper resting on his crossed knee. We talk about my willingness to do some exposure work - speaking of which I am regretting having worn such a revealing top. I sit well back when I realise and try surreptitiously to pull the neckline up. He doesn't seem to notice, or is deliberately ignoring me. I want to touch things in the room before I lose my nerve; he seems to have done his homework for once and suggests that as I had difficulties touching the table last week, how about me touching the top of the table at the other end of the room near the window. I do this once and return to my seat, heart

beating faster. Anxiety does its mountain peak stuff, then virtually drops away. The next time, he walks there with me, it seems a long way away.

'Keep your hands on the table this time Undine.'

'I can't'

'You can, look,' he kneels next to me and places his hands on the wood. I kneel too.

'It's awful,'

'Which word could you use instead, because things could be worse couldn't they?'

'I'm not sure they could.' It's as though my head is a steel basin being scoured with an industrial wire sponge.

'Keep your hands on the table, good girl. Keep breathing!'

'I find this very difficult.' English Understatement, plus I don't like being called a 'good girl'.

'I'm sure you do, don't let go. Move your hands around, Undine.'

I'm vaguely aware, above the shock and din in my head, that Alexander has stood up again. I stand slowly, my hands obediently pressed flat on the rough wood. He seems to be moving behind me, suddenly I feel the whole length of his body pushed hard against mine. I can't speak, I struggle but he clamps his hands over mine, he is bending my body slowly down towards the surface. If we fall onto the table something terrible will happen. It's ludicrous and embarrassing.

'You wanted this to happen, why wear that top otherwise?' he murmers triumphantly in my ear. I shake my head, I want to tell him it's a mistake. I try and twist to bite his arm, he laughs. When I kick backwards, he trips me forward. Darkness enfolds us as we mutely struggle.

I'm straining to speak, I have to because of Marius, if something happens it's my fault. But no sounds come out, just harsh panting.

'Undine,' he is saying now in my ear.

'Bubbles!'

I open my eyes with an effort. Marius is shaking my arm and staring at me, 'Wake up Bubbles, you kicked me!'

'Sorry,' I murmer groggily, trying to open my eyes properly, the chimera begins to fade in the dawn light. My heart is thumping painfully. The sheer relief that it was just a dream washes over me.

'You kept shouting "Alex", what were you dreaming about?

'It was horrible,'
'It didn't sound that horrible.' I'm alerted by a new note in his voice. Marius, jealous?
'Well it was. I'm so tired,' I pull weakly at the sheet twisted round me and reach to pull my pillow off the floor, 'I have to sleep now.' I kiss Marius's forearm which is the nearest part of him and instantly slide back into oblivion.

****

Gabriel

I think it was Bertrand Russell who said that the time you enjoy wasting is not wasted time: a man after my own heart. I'm lying on the sun chair on the deck, enjoying the Indian Summer rays, out of view of the denizens of the bank, cold beer on the table within reach. I'm ecstatic today not just because of this blissful idleness, but because Torquil admitted that Bubbles rang just before he went on holiday. He apologised so much for forgetting to tell me at the time, that I wasn't able to be angry with him. Anyway, it was most enjoyable telling him that it's been raining eels. Last night I found a long, fat, dead Eel on the deck when I got home from the hospital, it was a horrible sight. Decomposing, its tiny eyes were dry and innards had belched out from a split in the vast brown leathery skin. A Heron must have dropped it from the skies.

I looked across at the parasol suspended over the table and blurred my vision so that the central pole vanished. If one could invent floating sun-shades that moved with the sun to keep the object perfectly shaded ... That reminds me, I should put cream on Camberwell's ears, they're prone to sunburn. I'll do it in a minute, I can't be bothered to find the gauntlets. Anyway he's lying stretched out in the shade next to me at the moment, sensible cat.

All would continue to be bliss, if Torquil would stop repeatedly droning the first verse of the hymn, 'Eternal Father, strong to save'. In the old days, he'd have been frog-marched off the end of a plank. Trouble is, I can't say anything, because he's obviously indulging in wishful thinking: his parents arrive at four o'clock in honour of Torquil's birthday and his father is as substantial as a nasturtium. Torquil sprang the unexpected Royal Visit on me on Thursday when we'd had a particularly busy day on the MRI Unit. He arrived back late in the evening, having not visited *The Ark* for several days due to his rampant socialising. He inadvertently woke my pal Linda who was sleeping on the sofa rather than travel back to New Cross so late. He begged me not to let on that *The Ark* wasn't his place, heaven knows what he's told his parents, apparently I'm the lodger. They still seem to have no idea that Torquil's gay. I met his twin brother once: he's the heterosexual soul of convention.

Torquil seems really miserable today, I don't think it's just to do with his mother. However if he's made the bed (mine) for his parents once, he's made it several times and moved round it tweaking the pillows and duvet cover, as well as dusting and positioning everything else on the boat, until watching him became so painful that I had to go outside. He's out here now, tapping the feather duster on the railing to knock off a cobweb.
'You don't understand Gabriel, she's got a castrating gaze.'
He turned mournful long-lashed eyes on me.
'What?' I asked, startled.
'Not castrating gays, Silly, gaze.' Well, that accounts for a lot. She's successfully emasculated her son and husband, not to mention their two dogs.
'And she always makes beds with ironed sheets and the pillow cases facing the same way and hospital corners and everything is always in its same place and is shiny and immaculate.'
Anal cow. 'Torq, hey, it's okay. Have a drink.'
'No, that'll make it worse.'
'It doesn't matter what the boat looks like, so long as it isn't knee-deep in cockroaches and reeking of rot. I bet people would rather come here and relax, than sit on the edge of your mum's chairs clutching coffee cups while she brushes under their feet.'
'Mmm,' he didn't look convinced, but at least less agitated.
'I bet she's saying to your dad, does my make-up look all right? Do you think he'll like the cake we bought?'
'I won't, she always brings Battenburg!'

'That's better. Now make us a cup of tea if you can bear to sully the kitchen.'
He gave me a grateful smile and vanished indoors.

I can't stand Torquil's mother: she's an egocentric bully. I only said I'd stay around to give him moral support. Makes me realise how lucky I am with my family: we're not madly demonstrative, but if something happens we help each other, and we enjoy spending time together. I'm the youngest brother, there are three of us boys. My Mum and Dad are still contented together, unlike the parents of a lot of my friends it seems. A lot of Mums seem to be unhappy and chafing at the bit, a couple of them have broken free now the children are off their hands and moved on to pastures new. It must take some nerve to do that when you're fifty. I hope when I find the right person it lasts for ever – but I guess everyone wishes for that.

Torquil is always upset after his encounters with his parents. Unusually for her, this time his mother half-heartedly tried to prepare him for an unpleasant surprise. 'Daddy helped me with your card, but he got a bit muddled,' she whispered loudly. Torquil's father pretended to be deaf. Sure enough, the original name on the envelope was encrusted with a guano layer of Tippex and Torquil's name imprinted messily on top. Inside the card it said 'Happy Birthday Ronald, we love you to bits, lots of love and kisses, Mummy and Daddy xxx'.
Torquil looking wretched said bravely: 'You've given me the wrong card, you'd better take it back,' and tried to give it to Daphne, where she sat fanning herself on the sofa. The cats sat in an aggrieved semi-circle round her plump legs because she'd usurped their favourite seat.
'Oh no dear, Daddy and I chose it especially for you.' It had a picture of a smiling cartoon golfer in a checked sweater on the front. Why the hell didn't they just buy him another card? No wonder Torquil's got low self-esteem. I quietly slid away towards the kitchen, ostensibly to cut up the Battenburg - and got jammed in the sitting-room doorway with Torquil, who'd had the same idea.

It was difficult housing Ron Senior and Daphne as the boat is rather chaotic at present due to the renovation work on the kitchen and hold. Also they are 60+ and had to clamber over their suitcases to get into bed. How much luggage do they need to visit their two sons for a few days? Luckily they were too cowardly to clamber down the steep ladder into the hold and see Torquil's inflatable mattress on a sea of chipboard down there, which is where I slept in the end – Torquil sulkily slept in his sleeping bag on chipboard in another part of the hold. Unfortunately this morning, at seven o'clock, they yodelled down the ladder that other stuff they'd left in their Vauxhall, parked outside the Trust House, had been stolen. They were just setting off to drive to Ronald Junior's: apparently he's something approved-of in retailing. Would it be all right if they helped themselves to a teensy bit of toast? At which point I heard Torquil scuttling speedily up the iron ladder, as he'd bought enough breakfast for a buffet at the Waldorf.

****

Bubbles

The Anxiety Log hit 9 and 10 on the day that I left my friend Christie's flat near Oxford; I hoped my usual 'departure' nervousness wouldn't happen this visit, that the work with Alexander might be having more effect. I had to walk through a long city subway beneath a motorway at sunset. I was already tense, having been awake since dawn worrying about such things as, and fighting the temptation to, scratch words on the bed frame of the spare room. I was equally fearful that I'd left something under the bed (which entailed crawling around the floor obsessively inspecting wads of ancient dust), or whether I had marked the door, door handle … The list went on and on, but I don't think Christie noticed much, I masked my unacceptable anxiety with humour.

I was aware that although I was relaxed as I entered the long blue-tiled noisy tunnel, registering the graffiti-gilded bricks, angular autobiographical tags, swirling litter and piercing whiffs of urine, that soon I would be terrified as to whether I was leaving a mark on the place, perhaps by scraping my

shoe on the concrete floor. Running through the passage-
way might have solved it, but I was too weighed down by my
holdall. Darkness fell as I stood rigid, scarcely breathing, for
a long time in the filthy surroundings, clutching my bag and
trying to make sense of marks on the dimly-lit walls. Trapped
in my cerebral straitjacket.

****

Therapy Session

I related my panic in the subway to Alex, as an example of the
way in which I feel helpless to prevent the debilitating
accretion of anxiety and fear.
'Imagine that you are with a child who is walking through the
subway with you. This child does what you do, and keeps
checking things. What would you say to them, as an adult?'
'I don't have much experience of being with children. I'm not
very kind to children.'
Why did I say that? I knew why, it was a throwback to the
way I was in the past with my brother. I try to be nice to
children nowadays, and most of them seem to like me,
although I am scared of being around them in case I hurt
them.
'Sorry Alexander, what were you asking me?'
'What might you say to the child, as a kind adult?'
'I could say to him, let's have a look together at what you've
written?'
'Yes - let's call this child 'Little Undine','
'Oh, it's me, I hadn't taken that on board.' But Grania did
dress me in boy's shoes and often deny my femininity. I
wanted to be a frilly little girl, this was forbidden so I
obediently acted the muddy tomboy. Adults often mistook me
for a boy.
Ax was waiting, eyes watchful. I was aware that I was leaning
forward in my seat; he was leaning back.
'What else might you say?'
It felt like sums lessons at Primary School; I remembered
enjoying inscribing the numbers in my best writing with a
sharp pencil onto the bright white lined pages. But then I
couldn't get the right answer however hard I tried, and the

pencil would blunt and the page would become grey and marred by rubbings-out.

'Don't be silly?'

'No, that's critical adult.'

So what's the right answer?!

'I've said this before, but that's akin to the child sitting in a chair in the corner of an empty room, and the adult coming in, shouting 'No!' and then leaving, slamming the door. Bang!'

'You haven't told me that before.'

'Well, it's an analogy I often use. You are being empathic towards this child, rationally compassionate.'

'Isn't that a paradox? I mean, a mixture of logic and emotion? I thought to empathise is to have personal experience of something. You don't understand what it is like to have OCD, and never will!'

I hadn't realised how much resentment had been building up until it burst out of my mouth in a cartoon bubble filled with vitriol. Ax makes money and gains prestige from my distress. Does that compensate for help that he dispenses to vulnerable people, albeit sometimes accidentally?

'No, I don't know what it's like. Although, I think I have had a taste.'

Oh really? Alexander is sitting forward now, inappropriately excited and happy.

'During a session with a patient, I suddenly thought I might have left a cigarette burning back at the basement. I couldn't remember stubbing it out. I had to think very quickly through my normal pattern of behaviour. Would I have left a cigarette burning? I had to think through each step very quickly as I couldn't break up a session to return home and check.' He chatters on: '.... and so I worked out that I would never leave a cigarette burning.'

Sorry, you don't get membership or even admission to this exclusive club, Mate. I lean back and study the high white plaster cornicing. Alexander doesn't understand OCD emotionally, how could he? He's in a foreign country and should realise that he doesn't speak the language.

....

'I think I know where this fear of touching things comes from: Grania was always telling me not to touch things. Once in a shop together, a rare event, I remember she kept reiterating: "Don't touch anything Undine or you'll get a good hiding." But it wasn't mainly due to that, and I haven't told Alex so. Now I'm worried, and I can't access compassion towards myself without his permission. It's totally caught up with what I remember doing to my brother. Because I don't remember having this particular fear of indenting words onto things through touch, before that.

Fear of deliberately killing someone by touching them or making them jump when they have a weak heart, yes, or saying something that would bring the four beings of the apocalypse galloping, or of removing indispensable medication, or by causing broken glass to fall in someone's beer (that made working in a pub very difficult) or by dropping some devastating lie I'd written, or by any manner of other ingenious means - but not the putting of words onto things, in this particular incapacitating way.

OCD is a malevolent condition: you trick it into leaving you alone one way and it gets you another.

'What if you ask, "What are the chances that I touched this?"' Ax says.
'That doesn't mean anything to me... I could suggest to the child, Little Undine, that we touch the tunnel wall?'
'Yes, that's right!'
He looks relieved, I think he was beginning to give up.

****

Bubbles

Ax saying I have to build up a bank of compassion. I immediately hit a major problem with that: I don't feel I deserve one. I remember talking to a woman at a party, who, disconcertingly, turned out to be a therapist. She said that a belief of being non-deserving poisons everything. Perhaps I feel like this again because I haven't told Ax the bad thing I did to William. But Ax knows I did something. He doesn't take it very seriously though, which throws up interesting speculation about his attention span, or his memory of the rest of my session soliloquies.

I need to catch the escalating anxiety too, recognise it, which can be difficult. The techni-coloured OCD world is so fast, it jerks you up, spins like a fairground wall of death, and dumps you sickeningly hard, anxious and disorientated, with a burden of checking. Yanked back helplessly again and again, until staring and catatonic, but with my mind in a maelstrom.

Emotional suffering, abstract crap that it is. So many tears. So much clear liquid, enough to drown in. One therapist said pragmatically when I was on the rack with guilt about Grania's sad life: 'What point is there in two people suffering, instead of one?'
My friend Jo said, and I knew this at a deep level but had only once mentally addressed it, 'Your step-mother's jealous of you'.
A tough aspect to deal with: being told and perceived all the time as privileged and lucky, and feeling so full of dread. So much guilt for so many years, and later, when the inner numbness began painfully to thaw it felt similar to being Grandad, who had a small farm, coming in from milking outside in the black freezing dawn and seeing tears of pain on his averted face in front of the stove as his red hands thawed. My emotions are thawing.

When I feel so low there's no point in me beginning a new relationship with Gabriel. Sure, I could do my old thing of using sex as distraction from my thoughts, but it would hurt Gabriel a lot. I must be becoming more responsible. Gabriel seems really kind and I already like him, as well as finding him very attractive. Somehow, around him I feel able to be myself, a rare state, but I'd also have to tell him eventually what I'd done. What if he rejected me? I can't risk it.
I'll text him on his mobile and put a stop to any relationship before it starts. I'll somehow resist taking taking a ride on this particular roller-coaster.

****

Therapy Session

Alex tried to make sense of my Anxiety Log, it was three weeks worth crammed onto a page, so covered the time I spent visiting Christie. The scores had rocketed when I left the house to stay with her too. They were worse than usual because I knew nobody else would be at the house while I was away, Chloris being in Wales, and Matilda living it up in Spain with Dion. Well, except Matilda's friend, who's feeding Elvis. It took me over three-quarters of an hour to get out of the front door of Einstein Road, by the time I'd checked repeatedly that taps were off, iron was off, heaters were off, cooker was off, that sink plugs weren't in plugholes, lights were off, that the lavatory wouldn't overflow, that I hadn't shut Elvis in a door, that certain plugs were out of sockets, that I'd shut the fridge properly.... I was a nervous wreck. At this rate I'll be housebound again, unless it's like homeopathy where the condition might get worse before it gets better, I certainly hope so. Alex suggested I tick each room off on a sheet when I've checked it once, but I still have a problem using pens, so that wasn't very helpful. I'd also had a panic attack in the Library …

We could tackle this two ways, Alex interrupted eventually. We could do it quite intensively, but we need to practice talking compassionately to the 'small person' inside and not have too long a gap between the appointments.
He suddenly laughed: ' I can see dawning panic in your eyes at the thought of exposure techniques.' I was still trying to understand everything he was saying; the glass wall of panic had seamlessly and powerfully risen, cutting me off from comprehension. Anyway I relaxed, and said: 'You'd probably need a suit of armour, but what do you think of the idea of tackling the rituals intensively in three sessions on consecutive days?' (Marius has been doing a lot of business.) Alex said that would be all right, but to do it every other day, as every day was too much and the process needed time to settle down in between.

Homework is to fight avoidance behaviour, so I guess I'll have to stand as close as I can manage to counters in shops and the Bank, even touch them. It's depressing becoming aware of how much avoidance behaviour I perform in small ways - as well as realising that I've got a ritual list like a Telephobic Directory.

On the positive side, the aversion therapy seems to be working, slightly. I am beginning to understand that being an anxious person means I worry about things that other don't. That I suppress my anxious side because it was forbidden by Grania at home, and she mustn't be upset. But that was at the expense of me. Other people are sometimes more sympathetic, everyone is different. It's all right to for me to be nervous, to have OCD. Lots of people are highly-strung or have rituals, and their families are loving, humorous and supportive. Funny how long it took for that realisation to take hold. If I could use all the strength I previously used to conceal my condition and to prove that I was superwoman, to just do the things I enjoy without having to prove anything, how will my life change? And I'm beginning to realise that if I think the house is going to burn down if I don't check that the iron is off, someone else would cheerfully think it won't burn down, I'll take the risk and go down the pub. In other words, be gentle towards themselves.

....

Be that as it may, two long days later I texted Gabriel from Matilda's 'phone, saying I couldn't meet on Wednesday and had to be out of London for a while. I don't know how I managed it, but I'm frightened too of what Marius might do if he found out I was meeting Gabriel. He's becoming scary. I couldn't face seeing Gabriel at work, in case I weakened, so I managed to ring Vic and give in my notice. He was nice about me stopping the job immediately, perhaps because I said Juliet would be able to take over. She wants to be a silver statue rather than a gold one, but Vic didn't seem to mind. I'll have to go and sign on. I felt so low that evening, I cried myself to sleep.

****

Torquil

Yesterday was a haze of jumbled impressions. Heart racing, aftermath of stuff we did in the early hours after the club. My nipples really hurt, I think they are burnt from the amyl nitrate Gavin put on them. He gently taped little Mr Men plasters over them for me this morning, which helped. Gavin and I braved Ken High Street for some jeans this afternoon. Hopeless. He ended up with socks, plus a top that turned out to be too tight. Galvin sulkily said he didn't want to look like Batman and won't wear the T-shirt or take it back. I'll SMS him to finish it between us. I don't use abbreviations texting on the mobile when I don't want to see someone any more, just to be sure that they get the message. Anyway, it's only polite.

Poor Gabriel, he's so upset. That Bubbles is a right bitch. I won't say, but I told him so. I didn't like the way she was so abrupt to me that time she rang his mobile and I picked up.

****

Gabriel

I'm really miserable, I feel a right prat. Bubbles has sent a text saying she doesn't want to meet up. Chucked before I start, how bad is that!

'Would you prefer Evian or beer, Monsieur?' Torquil's being a good mate, very solicitous. For two euros he'd tell me there are plenty more fish in the river. Under his sympathy though, I sense satisfaction, or perhaps it's relief. If Bubbles was around permanently, he'd have to find somewhere else to stay.

Torquil is reluctant to sit down; I was getting worried about him, so he divulged that he's had a full wax treatment called Back and Sac. It makes my scrotum shrivel just to contemplate, he won't be using the exfoliating tub for a while. I think Torq's a bit of a masochist on the QT, well I know he is, with his small crosses of Elastoplast on his chest. Lucky he's got nipples or the plasters would just slide off, he's always

waxing. He's admitted he's been experimenting recently but got too scared, which has abruptly curbed his curiosity. Apparently it's all about power, and to stop whatever's going on when it's getting excruciating, you have to shriek some pre-arranged unlikely word. 'Stop' doesn't mean anything in those situations, so you arrange something like 'Anglesey' or 'calamine warthog'.
I don't understand how you can get fun out of it myself, merely being in love is mind-blowing and painful enough.

Bubbles is beautiful, but appearance *per se* doesn't matter. I've been out with people who are witty, intelligent, stunning, you name it, who aroused as much romantic interest in me – and probably vice-versa – as being tapped on the shoulder with a dead mackerel. You need the cerebral click, so that the world lights up when you see their profile or the way they walk.

Torquil suddenly seems very keen on me accompanying him to a party next month. Something in his manner's odd, so I checked if it was a heterosexual party, but he was evasive. Oh well, Torq knew the score, long ago.

****

Bubbles

Bubbles was sitting on the sofa in the sitting-room at Einstein Road. Since she and Matilda had washed the curtains and cleaned the windows, the room was much lighter. The brightness even spread through to the kitchen area which Matilda and Chloris had scrubbed out the previous week, everyone who came round remarked on the improvement. Chloris was going to buy white paint for the hall. Bubbles was currently staring vacantly at the 'Jobs Vacant' section in the *Ham & High*. Waitress... Typist...Shop assistant... Assistant to Interior Designer. She looked again, with more interest. No formal qualifications necessary, but ability to draw well, personable, enthusiastic, training on the job, NW3. She could do that, she could even cycle to work! Her shoulders sagged: what was the point? She probably wouldn't get it.

'Buy a lottery ticket you schmuck!' The punchline of a joke Finn had told them in the 'Hawley Arms' recurred. A man prays fervently to the Lord to win the Lottery, The first week he doesn't win, nor the second week, nor the third... She smiled. All right then. Bubbles sat back more comfortably on the sofa, and reluctantly tapped the number into the phone. While she listened to the ringing tone at the other end of the line, she tried to breathe deeply as Ax had taught her. In for the count of five, out for the count of ten. In... out, slower now-
'Good morning, 'Bon Idée Designs'!' A jubilant voice. Bubbles hyper-ventilated: 'Hello, I mean good morning, I'm ringing about your job, um your vacancy, advertisement-'

****

Gabriel

The seagulls outside the boat sound unnervingly like babies crying. The weather must be stormy at sea, there are so many of them. A cormorant has just flown past the window, dark against the grey lace of winter trees on the far bank. It's monochrome and freezing out there. The river swirls fast past the boat. I'm here alone, even the cats are nowhere to be seen, probably snugly curled up under the bed. I see people jog past on the towpath all the time, from five thirty in the morning to eleven at night, even at this time of year. On a more optimistic note, Autumn's the start of nature's cycle even though Winter's inexorably looming. At least I've got the multi-fuel stove this year. I used to wonder what the joggers were running from, or to. Now I reckon they're running away from their thoughts, themselves and their lives. I know there are millions of other women out there, but none like Bubbles. When I went to the Mall, there was a different girl under silver paint. During her break I asked her where Bubbles was, but she didn't know.

I wonder if in future there'll be J G Ballard-type scenarios being played out here: fortressed properties all along the Thames in London. There'd be no access to the river for anyone else, so there'd be no boats on it. In fact the river wouldn't be used at all. It would become little more than a trickle anyway, due to global warming. Then there'd be a rumour, say, that someone had pissed in it, from the South side, and that would be insult enough to start people firing guns, sniping at anyone they saw outside on the opposite bank. A civil war, north versus south London... I'm probably thinking like this because I'm depressed.

There's a fat red millionaire called Waddle, pushing fifty, who lives in a flat on the bank. He has a succession of cloned Lolita girlfriends. They're 'past it' as far as he's concerned, when they celebrate their eighteenth birthday. I've heard him boasting in *Pissed Up!* – and he was. I think it was his hawk-faced, leathery ex-wife on the alimony warpath yesterday, who kept trying to manoeuvre into my parking space. Unfortunately I was in it at the time, moodily mending a bike puncture. I resignedly indicated the large sign saying 'resurved for the Arc' - Alison having employed a dyslexic sign painter – before Leather-Face almost succeeded in running me down. When I asked her why she was giving herself bad kharma over a car space she wasn't entitled to use anyway, she furiously revved backwards and ripped the edge of her Jeep tyre open on one of the bollards. What goes around, comes around, I muttered within hearing while she was ringing the AA. She was also very abusive when I suggested she take up cycling, emphasising how it slims the legs down. I know, it isn't big and it isn't clever (as I overheard Dan saying to his young nephew, who had just been caught swearing) but it cheered me up.

****

Therapy Session

'I've applied for another job, as an Interior Designer's Assistant,'
'Yes?' Alexander couldn't sound less interested.
I've realised: I become upset by Alex when he suddenly reverts from our polite, friendly, 'intimate', relationship to one of a distant professional. It feels as though a spell is broken, a safe bubble burst and icy air howls in. I guess that all

psychotherapeutic relationships are intimate to a degree? But perhaps there are two spells: one is the safe, flexible, cosy one, the other tilts my world, disorientating and distressing me inordinately. I suppose that when Alexander suddenly switches off the charm and displays his genuine indifference to my life, it evokes Grania's attitude. I need to strengthen my identity, exercise the atrophied 'me' muscle, so that I stop being so dependent on Alexander. Which goes for everyone else. Then I'd be up to utilising Alexander's inconsistent behaviour, to finally deal with Grania's hurtful long-term lack of interest in me and my life.

'How would you feel about writing something now?'
'Right,' I could feel the blood draining from my face, but I'm here to tackle the fear. Could be a jingle for bungee jumping, I'm here to conquer the fear, da de da de da, SPLAT. He handed me a pen which I held as gingerly as I would a bomb, you couldn't retract the biro point. For two pins I'd have hurled it away from me across the room.
'Quickly,' I muttered. I thought my face would shatter with tension.
'Can you manage another minute?'
'I'm not sure,'
He's staring at me, I can feel it as I stare at the pen point in the air, two centimetres beyond the end of my fingers. You cannot write on air with a biro. Slowly he hands me two sheets of paper, and worse, a file to rest them on. I might write something bad on it, it'll get indented.
'Breathe Undine.'
I hadn't realised I was holding my breath. My shoulders sag, I breathe rapidly. Clumsily, due to holding the pen in the air, I hold the pages as lightly as possible and rapidly drop them onto the file on my lap.
'I can't manage, Alexander.'
'Yes, you can, another few seconds?'
'No!'
'All right, now just write, about anything you like, enjoy the experience if you can, the smooth paper, the creativity.' I snorted shakily, 'I'll tell you when to stop.'
'Please give me a subject, so that I can think about that.'
'All right,' he looks at a loss, imagination is obviously not his forté. 'How about, that bird outside on the window sill.'

So I wrote about the bird, which flew away, writing as fast as I could so that I didn't get caught up in correcting and worrying about what I'd written. The handwriting of course was ugly, but that didn't matter. Just as I was beginning to slow after a couple of minutes, and to obsessively change a letter, an 'a' it was, Alex told me to stop.

He took the piece of paper, folded it neatly into quarters and put it in his back pocket. I stared at him.

'How do you feel on a scale of 1-10?' I don't know, it's not relevant.

'It's going up, fast.' It rocketed up to 8 as the page remained in his jeans pocket, then we talked of other things and I sort of forgot it.

'So what your anxiety level now?' Alex asked ten minutes later.

'Three? But when you ask, it triggers it to rise.'

'Do you want to try and write something else?'

'I don't know.'

'You're doing brilliantly.'

This time I chose the subject, and wrote a short love poem about Peter Pan, just for the hell of it. Alex secreted that in the same manner in another pocket.

After that I was utterly exhausted. I had a mental rest until the end of the session while he wrote up notes, of other patients I think, but I couldn't think any more. It didn't occur to me to ask Alex for the pages back to check. I must have subconsciously decided to do things the hard way. Same old pattern.

What struck me, when I dared to look at the form I filled in months ago now for Alex,

s a) a spelling mistake (me!) and b) how little of it I'd actually completed. I was fulfilling my usual pattern of behaviour of not engaging totally with things.

Note the 'was', I'm getting better.

****

Romance

True to her word, Naomi phoned Ursula on Monday morning.
'Ursula, congratulations, I'd like to offer you the job.'

*Ursula thanked her and Naomi caught the elation in her voice.
'You were the best person I saw, by far,' she said warmly. 'I'll
send you the contract to sign today. Would you like to start
next Monday, then I can show you the ropes for a week
before I leave?'
'Yes,' agreed Ursula happily.
'Oh and do you have the exact dates of the week you're going
ski-ing next month? Sophie is willing to cover then.'
Ursula told her that she probably wouldn't be going now, and
with mutual good wishes they rang off.
Ali tried to smile when he saw her bounce into the kitchen
humming.
'Was that the job?'
'Sorry Ali, yes it was,' she admitted.
'Congratulations,' he said glumly.
Ursula suddenly thought, what am I apologising for? He
hasn't behaved well. Ali shamefacedly remembered the
same.
'Good for you,' he said more warmly. 'Come on, let's go to
Julie's Wine Bar - I know you don't drink but I do.*

*As the plane took off, gusts of snowflakes swirled in the
gloom outside the window. Ursula hadn't really minded the
weather; she had been manageress at Dreams for a month
now, and was thoroughly enjoying it. As Naomi had
promised, Sophie was fun to work with. Ursula felt her
confidence increasing daily as she chose stock, liaised with
clients and arranged the window displays. A few of her
previous clients from Clouds had already transferred their
patronage to her new workplace - Ursula was relieved that
Celia Huysman wasn't among them - and were very
complimentary about the shop. They were also flattering, she
felt, about her own more attractive appearance. Against her
will, she remembered the way Celia's eyes had lit up at the
sight of Anthony. They made a good pair, both horrible, she
thought deliberately childishly. But she couldn't help feeling a
pang; why did she have to find him so attractive?
Unconsciously she turned her plastic glass of mineral water
round and round between slim fingers. Her wedding ring
caught the light. Ali had eventually managed to persuade her
to wear it again. '- Just until you move out of the flat, Ursula,'
his pleading voice sounded again in her ears. Why not?*

She'd thought, it's not going to make any difference to anything.

The coach from the airport climbed tortuously along narrow zig-zagging mountain roads through the cold darkness towards the resort. Towering banks of snow edging the road were picked out fretfully in the bus's headlights, before falling back into dark shadow. An occasional car, driven recklessly fast, sloshed past them on the way down. At last, the crowded coach stopped in a small forecourt, and they saw with relief the bright neon sign on the front of a wooden three-storey hotel. It was bitterly cold. Ursula looked up standing beside the bus. They seemed surrounded by mountains, it felt comforting. A bright silver moon cast shadows on the icy snow. She and Ali followed the other guests carefully across the gritty snow into the brightly-lit warm foyer.

In the morning Ursula woke and stretched quietly, so as not to wake Ali in the other bed. She showered and dressed in the bathroom, adding a warm soft red polo-necked jumper beneath her new white ski suit. As she re-emerged, she pulled the curtains back quietly and gasped at the beauty of the dazzling snowy landscape sloping up and away outside their chalet. In the distance she could see cable cars. Nearer the hotel was the drag lift, wending it's way off up the mountain. A few early skiers were astride the metal poles, being pulled up the slope. A translucent icicle, as thick as her arm, hung outside the window tapering down from wooden eaves above. The sky reminded Ursula of the glorious cerulean blue in her water-colour box. She was glad she had brought her paints with her, it had been a last minute impulse. Perhaps this afternoon she could go up in one of those bubble-shaped cable cars, and sit outside the cafe Ali had told her about at the top. She could sunbathe and do some preliminary sketches. But first she had ski class this morning, Ursula thought excitedly. Ali was still soundly sleeping, so she left a note saying she had gone to breakfast, and quietly let herself out into the warm corridor.

The class stood in an uneven line along the nursery slope. Every few minutes, tiny children on skis, hands clasped behind their backs, would fearlessly shoot past them down the mountain into the distance. The class smiled at each other: 'Tomorrow,' promised Luc, the bronzed French instructor, 'You will be doing that, also without your sticks'. The class groaned. However, by the end of the morning, Ursula could gently snow plough to a halt. Very hot, she pushed her thick plait back over her shoulder, and unzipped her suit almost to her waist.

The class disbanded amiably, and she made her way slowly to the cable car to meet Ali at the mountain-top cafe, as they'd arranged. Outside the wooden shed where the cars halted, Ursula bent down and removed her skis with difficulty. The bindings were quite stiff. She clumped up the wooden steps in her heavy ski boots, to join the queue. She stacked her skis in the holder on the outside of the car, and another woman climbed in after her. The small cable car swayed as it climbed higher suspended from the wire, another passed them noisily on the way down. The buildings of the ski resort became tiny below them, then disappeared behind a ridge.

She saw Ali sitting at one of the wooden bench tables outside the crowded cafe in the sunshine. He waved; proudly Ursula skied the small slope down towards the cafe. Too late, she realised she couldn't stop. Snow plough as she might, she inexorably slid on. Panicking, Ursula threw herself sideways, falling through shadow into a small drift of snow. Laughing helplessly, she tried to undo her skis, becoming gradually aware there was a pair of legs standing still in front of her. Looking up further, pushing her sunglasses up onto her head, she felt the smile freeze on her face. The man looking sardonically down at her, clad devastatingly in a professionally black ski suit, with Varnier sunglasses slung round his neck, was Anthony. Ursula gaped at him speechlessly.
'You!' he said. Abruptly he extended a hand down towards her. She pretended not to see it and thrashed around in the snow trying to rise.
'Take hold Ursula, I won't bite!' he said impatiently. Her senses jumped as he spoke her name, he pulled her to her feet with ease. The skis slid treacherously as she pulled her hand quickly away, as she fought for balance she found herself sliding slowly towards him. Easily he put her at arms'

*length, his hands resting casually on her narrow waist. His
severe expression relaxed into a smile. 'Steady' his deep
voice said caressingly as his eyes flicked over her body.
Returning to her face, he raised his eyebrows at her indignant
expression.
'I...I don't stare at you' she blurted out suddenly.
'You do actually, but I don't happen to mind' he rejoined
infuriatingly. His eyes narrowed with an amused interest.
'When we met in Barkers, you were wearing rather less. So
why do you mind me looking at you now?' he asked softly.
'That was different,' she said weakly. She felt mesmerised.
Seemingly suddenly bored with baiting her, Anthony looked
away. Ursula wondered if he'd remembered she was married.*

****

Undine

In the textbook it says that 'the effective behavioural treatment
of OCD requires intensive intervention [that word has
unpleasant echoes] on the part of the therapist and and
strong motivation on the part of the patient.'
Hey ho, well I think Alexander and I have just enough energy
and mutual forbearance between us to pull it off. I hope so.

Actually, it proved really difficult to obtain medical books
about OCD. I rang University College Hospital, the
Receptionist of which was courteously helpful. She
suggested I verify that their Rockefeller Library did actually
hold the books by checking their catalogue on the Internet
(Chloris did it for me at work). Sure enough, they only had
one of the five titles I'd managed to glean by ringing up an
OCD therapist, and that was out on loan for another three
weeks. When I'd asked Alex for information to help me to
research my condition, he'd made uncharacteristically vague
noises and didn't seem to want me to have the information. I
asked in a local bookshop and they could order one of the
titles for me, but I couldn't afford the book at £38.

I broached the local Library. Tensely holding the list of titles, I
asked the tanned Antipodean behind the information desk in a

whisper if she had *Treatment Plans and Interventions for
Depression & Anxiety Disorders.*
'What's thit agin?' she asked loudly enough to wake those
dozing limply on chairs in the Exercise and Beauty section.
'Treatment Plans for-'
I held the paper across the desk and pointed: 'That one.'
'She tapped, Treatment p.l.a.n.s. for ..... [pause] No, we
haven't got that. What are those others, you want me to
check?'
'Yes please, er, could you order me a copy of each book?'
'Sure, but it costs £1.50, it can take six to eight weeks.'
'Okay,' I murmered, rather dismayed.
'Yes, depends where we have to order it from, how far afield.
Let me just look.... Are you a student?'
'Er, no.' The Librarian caught herself staring at me strangely,
and looked back at the keyboard. She was probably checking
me for nervous tics.
'Haven't got that one, or that one.... Anxiety? Nah, it's
reserved for ages.'
On the last title: 'Oh yeah,' she bellowed cheerfully, 'We've
got 'Stop Obsessing.'
I ordered it. I hadn't realised how many anxious people
reside in NW5: it feels a very friendly place now.

I bravely 'phoned the Maudsley Hospital. A pleasant woman
put me through to the library at the Institute of Psychiatry, a
horrible woman tersely answered the phone: 'Library!' I
didn't know you could enunciate it with one syllable. I'd
written prompts on my reminder pad before I made the 'phone
call, now I read from it:
'Excuse me, I'm writing a book about Obsessive Compulsive
Disorder, do you have any books on the subject?'
'Yes, but they are not available to anyone who is not a
student or member of staff here.'
How does she know I'm not? Because I use three syllables?
'So I can't come in and refer to them?' I ad-libbed hopefully.
'No,' she said gleefully, putting the 'phone down.
I was incredulous: that's disgusting, keeping information from
people, especially vulnerable members of the public.

****

'I've been there of course. It is very grim, as almost everyone's suffering from Depression.' It's comments like these that stop me confiding in Alex. Poor depressives, seeing themselves mirrored in a resentful, sullen librarian who's letting the side down by not being a ray of sunshine.

When I related the story of the old bag to Finn in the 'Hawley Arms' on Saturday lunchtime (I've 'come out' to him about my OCD) he scoffed and said a Librarian's job wasn't stressful. 'Any job can be stressful, Finn,' I disagreed, timidly. 'Gah!' He is reassuringly stolid. You can feel his bolshie Irish genes alive and kicking beneath his deadpan exterior. 'I'm really fed-up. I wish I had enough money to go travelling, somewhere hot where I'd get a nice unhealthy sun-tan.' I said wistfully, staring into my lager. 'You are tanned.' 'Do you think so? I've been going swimming with Matilda at the Heath.' 'What happened about the job? You went for an interview didn't you?' 'Yes, I haven't heard anything yet. It's been a week, do you think I could ring them?' 'Sure, why not? You'll look keen.' I took another sip of sparkling mineral water with ice and lemon: de-toxing wasn't so bad if I pretended the fizzy rip-off was Cava. 'I know it's not quite the same, but I've got to brave the wilds of west London and deliver a mattress next Saturday. You can come along if you like,' Finn offered. 'Keep me company.' 'Okay, where?' 'Somewhere near the Hogarth Roundabout, you can navigate.'

****

Einstein Road

'At last! I thought you were avoiding me, I've had to keep speaking to the witch!' 'Chloris has been nice lately. She's all right when you get to know her.'

Marius snorted derisively and, slamming the front door behind him, followed Bubbles into the kitchen at Einstein Road. It was early Saturday evening. He collapsed noisily onto a chair and swung his heavy black boots up to rest on the kitchen table. Bubbles filled the kettle under the cold tap not looking at him.

'Give us a cuddle, babe,' he ordered. Bubbles avoided Marius's outstretched hands and plugged in the kettle. Reluctantly she stopped moving and leaned against the stone sink, out of reach, folding her arms around herself.

'What's going on darling?' He sounded genuinely bewildered, Bubbles had to remind herself that Marius only ever made an effort to be charming if he felt he was losing his hold over her.

'I told you, Marius, I've met someone else.'

'Well, you didn't expect me to take that seriously did you? You and I have been together quite a while, on and off.'

'I've met someone else, Marius.'

'Okay, okay. Saying he exists, who? Where?'

'Just a guy. A couple of weeks ago, in west London.'

'What, at your job?'

'No, maybe.'

'So that's me, just dropped,' he said bitterly, slamming his boots down onto the kitchen floor.

Bubbles flinched.

'All that money I've poured into your arty-farty therapy, hoping it would help us. Just down the drain.' Marius suddenly stood, his chair scraping loudly on the tiles.

'I'll pay you back.'

'Don't talk crap, when did you ever pay anyone back?' Marius was shouting furiously.

'Actually, Chloris leant me some money last month, and I've given her some back, from my statue job.' With surprise, Bubbles realised this was true.

'Right, you can repay that bitch, you give me what's mine!'

'You got yours dealing drugs, it's different.' Bubbles muttered.

'Are you threatening me? Because if you are-' Suddenly Marius was pressed hard against her, yanking her head painfully far back by her hair, gripping her throat murderously in his other fist, lifting her onto her toes. Bubbles couldn't breathe, his breath rasped against her face, the sink bruised her rigid back. Past his blurred head, the kitchen became misty.

'You fucking bitch.' The steel buttons on his jacket hurt her
ribs. She thought there was a flicker of bright light. In the
distance there was a loud clang, Marius's grip relaxed and he
fell away. There was another crash.
Released, Bubbles collapsed forward, gasping for air,
hanging onto the work surface.
'That'll teach him,' said Chloris with satisfaction, replacing her
Le Creuset frying pan on a hook above the cooker.
'Undine, are you all right?' Bubbles felt Chloris semi-lifting
her across to a chair. 'Come on, that's right.' Chloris
crouched beside her, rubbing her arm and staring into her
face as Bubbles struggled to breathe. Eventually Bubbles sat
back in the chair, she saw Chloris's hand put a glass of water
on the table beside her. She supposed she was in shock.
She could see Marius, lying splayed on the floor near her feet.
'Matt! Matilda!' Chloris had disappeared into the hall, could
be heard running up the stairs. An answering call came from
above, then there was a murmur of conversation, an
exclamation. Marius was beginning to stir, his eyes opened.
Bubbles looked at him mutely, terrified. She couldn't move.
Just then Matilda appeared, stared sympathetically at
Bubbles who felt embarrassed, then said 'Ready?' to Chloris.
She picked up Marius's feet while Chloris grabbed him under
the armpits. Together they hefted him through the doorway,
banging his shoulder hard against the architrave, and into the
hall. Bubbles heard the front door open, Marius say: 'Wha's
going on?' in a muzzy voice, then the heavy door slam. They
reappeared, dusting their hands, 'Better out than in,'
'Sure. I can't believe you did that Chloris!'
'Domestic violence makes my blood boil, I come across it
sometimes at work. It's nice to tackle it head-on for once.'
'And how!'
'Do you think he'll be all right?' Bubbles asked hoarsely. She
wanted to wash her neck where Marius had touched it, the
skin burned, she felt dirty.
'I don't know Undine, I don't really care, to tell the truth.'
'But it's my fault all this happened, if he dies or is injured it's
my fault,' Bubbles was suddenly crying helplessly, her throat
and eyes ached horribly.
'No,' She was aware that Matilda had her arm round her
shoulders.

'No it won't, it'll be mine,' said Chloris firmly. 'But the wicked always survive, unfortunately. Who wants some of my carrot cake?'

Bubbles and Matilda looked at Chloris respectfully: 'Yes please,' said Matilda, Bubbles nodded, shakily wiping her eyes.

'I'll just go and see if he needs a doctor, it'll make me feel better,' said Bubbles apologetically, getting up unsteadily. 'He's not there,' she said, closing the front door and slowly returning to the kitchen.

'Not dead yet then,' said Chloris briskly. She pushed the plunger down in the cafetiere, a smell of fresh coffee lightened the air. Bubbles gingerly touched the back of her head, she was scared to, wondering if Marius had wrenched out chunks of her hair. Her scalp felt tender, but normal. Matilda was busily laying out plates, cups, knives and napkins.

'Here Undine, have something to eat, take your mind off it. The sponge is really soft.' Chloris pushed the sliced cake gently towards her.

'Thanks,' Bubbles felt herself smiling at her friends as they sat round the table. 'Oh, you're so kind, I'm going to cry again.'

'That's all right - can you manage some coffee first?'

****

It was a beautiful autumnal day a fortnight later: 'What caused these?' Bubbles asked rashly, looking up at interesting ochre stains splashed across the van ceiling.

'Oh I reckon someone came hurtling through the windscreen in the past, bleeding profusely,' said Finn.

'Finn!'

He laughed comfortably, grinding gears, his gold earring glinted in the sunlight.

Bubbles was relieved she was wearing a white polo-neck that hid the faint bruises on her neck and back, and that her eyes were no longer bloodshot. She didn't want Finn to know what had happened with Marius, he would be sympathetic but indiscreet. As they revved up to fifty miles an hour along the Westway, the van rattled deafeningly. Bubbles craned round to peer into the cavernous back of the vehicle, the mattress was still slumped heavily against one of the metal walls, protected from the dusty floor by a sheet. Nothing appeared to be loose.

'It's the back bumper, up in the roof rack.'

'Oh, right.' Bubbles was really enjoying the journey, albeit relieved they'd got this far. Finn had not asked for many directions. The back step of the ancient blue Transit was a ridge of rust and the double doors were tied closed with a piece of orange rope. There was a strange musty smell in the cab, but plenty of leg-room and it was fun looking down on traffic for a change. Fin had thoughtfully given her a clean towel to sit on, Bubbles adjusted the broken seat belt over her shoulder to give an illusion of legality.

Council skyscrapers appeared on the Brentford horizon: the same ones as she'd passed on her first arrival in London eight years before. She remembered realising with shock that each light represented at least one person, like her in her bedsit. The number of tiny lights in one monolithic block alone had amazed her. Now they were trundling comfortably in the van towards the Hogarth Roundabout. Bubbles had always loathed this as an urban monstrosity on her rare bus journeys back to Oxford, and wondered who in hell would want to live here. To her surprise, they turned down a narrow road, then left along a pretty street, the van making heavy weather of the speed bumps. A pastoral cemetery appeared along one side, they skirted a small quiet roundabout, and parked in a modern development of three-storey flats.

'Hang on here a sec.' said Fin, pushing open his creaking door with difficulty, 'I'll just go and see if he's in, I don't want you having to heft that mattress again.'

Warmed by his consideration, Bubbles sat back and relaxed. All was silent, she cranked down her window. In front of the van was a large open area with an ornamental folly in the centre. Behind that appeared to be some sort of promenade. Bubbles clambered out of the van, stretched luxuriantly, and crossing the promenade, leant on black iron railings surveying the Thames with delight. Two swans floated one behind the other in the distance, before the one behind grew level with it's mate and they briefly appeared as one, before it sailed on ahead.

The tide was high, the water flowing fast beneath a long, wooden, ramp to her left. This led down to a pontoon where four large boats were moored. Bubbles pushed her sunglasses up onto her hair and raised her face to the bright wide sky, closing her eyes. The sun was warm on her face. 'Bubbles, want to come down?' She heard Fin's voice faintly, and squinted at the pontoon. He was looking up at her, and next to him was Gabriel. Bubbles felt light-headed, she grabbed at the railing.
'Coming,' she called unsteadily.
There was a hissing in her ears, the sunlight seemed dazzling. Nervously, she adjusted her sunglasses and made her way hesitantly along the ramp.
'Well hello...Bubbles.' said Gabriel meaningfully. He seemed calm and looked stern. Of course, he knew her as Bubbles: 'That's my nickname,' she said quickly.
'Do you two know each other?' asked Finn, surprised.
'Yes, we met when I was doing that statue job at Hammersmith,' she said. Bubbles couldn't stop staring at Gabriel. He folded his arms, he was wearing a navy fisherman's jumper and Chinos.
'I didn't realise it was your Futon,' she said.
'Otherwise you wouldn't have come?' he asked.
'Yes, I would... I don't know.' Suddenly unhappiness overwhelmed her, she stared down at her leather boots.
Finn was looking edgy: 'I'll let you two have a couple of minutes,' he muttered, and walked away as they protested.

'Gabriel...'
'What?'
'I really wanted to, you know, have a relationship with you, but I have a lot of problems...'
'You didn't give me the option of deciding whether I minded that, did you?'
'No. I'm sorry.'
There was a silence as he turned away and looked at the river, and she looked up at his profile. He was beautiful.
'I don't know if I could cope, being with someone...'
'I'm willing to give it a try if you are,' he said suddenly, turning back to look at her. The sun shone on his ash-blonde hair.
Everything fell silent, as though they were in a play.
'All right,' Bubbles said shakily, then burst into tears.

'Hey,' he said, reaching out a strong arm and pulling her to his chest. Gabriel cuddled her, gently rubbing my back, 'I don't usually have this effect on women I ask out,' he said ruefully.
'I'm sorry,' Bubbles blew her nose on his handkerchief.
'You don't have to apologise.'
'I'll wash it for you,' she said, indicating the damp handkerchief.
'Whatever... I don't know what you prefer to be called - Bubbles or Undine?' he asked, smiling.
'Undine, please – in fact Bubbles is a goner!'
He kisses thrillingly.
'Um, guys,' it was Finn, who seemed to have a bad cough. 'Do you want this Futon or what? It's just that I've got to get back to Camden to give Art a lift.'

Undine

After we'd all hefted the mattress which seemed to have a life of its own and no handles, down the ramp to the boat, we had a cup of tea. I noticed Gabriel wasn't limping any longer. Then Finn rose to go, I'd been dreading this. He said: 'Ready then?' to me and opened the front door. Reluctantly I reached for my sunglasses, I didn't want to leave. I was willing Gabriel to say something so that the relationship would carry on. As Finn stepped down on to the crates, Gabriel said hurriedly, looking at me: 'I've got two free tickets to Madame Butterfly at the Opera House for tonight, through work. I don't know if you enjoy that sort of music...?'
'I love it!' I blurted. I do too, but Gabriel could have offered me an evening at the local vets and still had the same ecstatic reaction.
'So am I going back on my own?' asked Finn with disappointment, but with the gossip light in his eye. It'd be all round Camden by tomorrow, Undine getting off with a virtual stranger and bringing her own mattress. Whatever happened I wasn't going to give in to my lustful urges and stay the night.
'Oh sorry Finn, but yes.'
'How come true romance doesn't happen for me every time I have something delivered?' We all laughed.
'Yes mate, but look on the bright side, you'll have room to pick up hitch-hikers now. Thanks for bringing the mattress, we'll go for a drink next week.' Gabriel's voice receded as he escorted Finn up the ramp.

****

Torquil

'Hi Sheila'
'Torquil! Long time no hear, how's it going?
'Great, well ...'
'Are you still living on the boat with Gabriel? I don't mean, with- Oh, you know.'
'Yes, but there's a bit of unwelcome change in the air.'
'Oh? Do tell.'
'Yes, not me. Though there is this lovely boy, Christopher, I'm working on him. I've agreed to go with him to do 'Crisis Open Christmas, it's working at homeless people's shelters. He does it every year.'

'You?!'

'What *do* you mean, saying it like that?'

'Judy Garland, yes, Mother Theresa, no - but good for you, Torq! He must be a hunk if you're giving up your Christmas.'

'Certainly is.'

'What a waste. What about all us desperate single women?' There was a pause.

'Is Gabriel seeing anyone?' Sheila couldn't help herself.

'Ah, that's partly why I'm ringing. There's this silly bint hanging around, called Undine.'

'Undine! What a name,' mocked Sheila with enjoyment.

'Yeah, lives up to it to, peroxided airhead by all accounts.'

'What, you haven't met her?'

'Not yet, it's a new development, but Gabriel's putty in her legendary. At this rate she'll be moving in.'

'Oh.'

'Why don't you pop over and cheer me up? You haven't seen the boat yet. If you can extricate Gabriel from her clutches at the same time, you'll be my friend for life.'

'I thought I already was.'

'Not if you don't use your magic womanly charms! Only joking. Seriously, I never understood why you and Gabriel never made it to the altar.'

'I wanted to, he had commitment-phobia.'

'Are you free Thursday evening?'

****

Undine

'Do you want me to come and meet you somewhere en route?'

'No, it's all right, thanks. The E3 'bus you said?'

'That's the one, right outside Turnham Green tube, if you're sure you want to do it that way instead of coming on the North London line?'

'Yes, I'm coming from town as I'm going shopping with Matilda first,'

'Right, see you around six then Darling.'

We rang off.

'Darling', Gabriel called me 'darling'. I skipped around the kitchen. I'd talked on the phone with him without having a panic attack and being tempted to say all sorts of stupid things.

I bored Matilda to death about Gabriel, while we were hunting for material for her at Berwick Street market. She seemed very pleased for me, which was fun, and keen to meet him. That's another thing: for once I'm not anxious about introducing an attractive new boyfriend to my girlfriends. Either I trust him or them more, or maybe myself.

....

As I trotted down the ramp, hoping I still looked pretty after all my efforts with cosmetics, hair-primping and flattering clothes – Gabriel came out onto the walkway and waved. 'I heard the gate close, and hoped it was you,' he said as I drew nearer. I felt suddenly shy, when I glanced at him he seemed to sense this and drew me into an embrace, kissing me warmly. We only stopped because someone moved nearby. We pulled apart. There was a scarily attractive auburn-haired girl, around my age, leaning over the railing on the boat deck: 'You must be Undine, Gabriel's told us all about you,' she said.
Gabriel looked annoyed and slightly shook his head, 'I haven't said a word, Undine. Aren't you supposed to be meeting Torquil, Sheila?'
She blushed slightly, 'I'll wait for him a bit longer, I don't know what's happened to him, must be something at work.'
'Torquil?' I asked, to try and lighten the atmosphere.
'Oh, he's a designer, of sorts, he shares the boat with me.'
'He's your tenant,' said the woman, 'Face up to it Gabriel, after all your Leftie beliefs, you're a landlord.'
'Waterlord actually.' Gabriel and I smiled. 'Anyway, let's get you indoors out of the cold, Undine.'
I followed him up the beer crates, Sheila leading the way into the sitting-room.

It seemed rather awkward, having a glass of wine with Sheila there. I noticed that the dining-table was laid for two, I hoped it was for Gabriel and I.

'How did I let you go?' Sheila said, deliberately laying her hand over his on the wine glass he handed to her. I was pleased to notice Gabriel pull his hand away so abruptly that the wine almost slopped over her lace sleeve. Sheila sat cross-legged on the sofa next to Gabriel revealing an expanse of slim brown legs and leaning forward whenever she spoke, in a low-cut top. She scarcely looked at me, sitting in a chair by the door, although Gabriel had offered to swap seats with me. Sheila addressed her remarks to Gabriel as though she was his girlfriend and they'd had a little tiff. After seeing her stroke his knee for the third time, I put down my empty glass and decided to leave.

'I have to get back now,'

'But you've only just come.' He looked distressed. 'I'll walk you to the Tube.'

'No, it's fine.'

'No, it's not. Sheila, I'm cooking a meal for Undine and I. I'm afraid there isn't enough food for three.'

'Well, do you mind if I wait for Torquil? I'll just sit over here and read a book, you won't know I'm here.'

Gabriel paused, obviously at a loss for what to say. I hated her.

'I'm going, thanks for the wine Gabriel.'

I grabbed my coat and hat, and hurried outside. As I breathlessly reached the gate, a hand reached round me to open it, making me jump. I turned, Gabriel was hurriedly pushing his other arm into his coat.

'I'm sorry about that Undine, I don't know why Sheila's here. Well, if we can't dislodge her, we'll go out. Do you like pub food, there's a good place along the bank a little way?'

So that's what we did, we escaped from Sheila and had a great evening. I haven't laughed so much for ages.

Later Gabriel said more soberly: 'I haven't seen her for years. She was a very tenacious ex-girlfriend.'

'She still is.'

'You've nothing to fear; I just wonder what she's playing at.' He looked grim.

As we walked back with our arms round each other along Chiswick Mall, avoiding tree branches and flotsam left on the road by the high tide, we chose our favourite mooring gardens. I couldn't decide between one with bronze dogs, or another with a huge sculpture of a pomegranate displayed on a lawn under a tree. Gabriel chose a wild unkempt garden brimming with plants and trees.

'That's what my allotment probably looks like at the moment, I haven't had time to go there for a couple of months, I'm still Temping at the hospital. I remember an old guy saying ominously when I first got it: 'The curse of allotments are young working people!''

Gabriel was very good at impersonating a grumpy old man, I hoped he would get another acting job soon.

'You're stopping work at the hospital in mid-January, aren't you? I know that's over three months away but you'll have time then to do the allotment, if by any chance you don't get an acting job straight away. You won't need much money for seeds and stuff, look here's free manure!'

'That's from the horses the police ride along here. That must be a lovely job.'

'You'll have a great job soon Gabriel, on television,' I hugged him. 'Have you any auditions lined up?'

'Actually I've just seen one for a vet …'

'I'm sure you'll get it,' I said devoutly.

'Bless you Undine,' Gabriel pulled me towards him and we kissed blissfully in the moonlight.

....

I don't know how I resisted the temptation to christen the new mattress, but I made it home last night on the last Tube, Gabriel smiling farewell at me from the platform as the train pulled out. When I finally let myself in at Einstein Road Chloris was still up, reading a magazine, she'd been out with a friend from work so we had a nightcap and I told her about Gabriel. When I mentioned Sheila, Chloris said: 'She sounds difficult,' wrinkling her forehead. 'It would take some nerve for her to behave like that when he didn't want her around.'

That sowed a seed of doubt in my Garden of Eden, but I cheered up by remembering how warm Gabriel had been towards me, and how cold towards her.

'Oh sorry Undine, I meant to say before, there's a message for you on the answerphone from Bon Idee Designs. I only heard the beginning, I left it for you.'

I played it back. It was the offer of an interview at the office in Hampstead. Chloris and I crowed with delight and had another small nightcap to celebrate. Bad things happen in threes, but so do good things, *c'est la vie*. Chloris and I gossiped and role-played the interview until two o'clock in the morning.

****

Romance

'Where are you staying?' he asked abruptly.
'At the Three Stars Hotel.'
'So are we!' he exclaimed, startled.
'We', the word reverberated in Ursula's head.
'Were you delayed from going up to Les Arcs 2000 too, by the avalanche?' he asked.
'No, we're staying there.'
'Anthony,' a female voice called. Startled, Ursula almost fell over as a female skier wheeled sharply to a halt beside them. Powdered snow sprayed Ursula's legs.

It was Celia. Looking unbelievably glamorous in a sea-green ski suit and dazzling white boots, white headband holding back thick auburn hair. She looked disinterestedly at Ursula, then her eyes suddenly sharpened with recognition.
'Hang on, aren't you... didn't you work at Clouds?' Now Celia's eyes incredulously raked Ursula's glossy hair and figure-hugging ski suit. Ursula in turn became aware that lumps of snow on her suit were melting. Her arms felt damp and her feet were cold; she shivered. Looking round she could see Ali was standing by his table. He was shading his eyes with his hand, looking across anxiously.
'Thank you for picking me up,' she said politely. Anthony smiled.
'No, I mean - well anyway, I must go. I'll get warm in the sun,' she floundered. Anthony's eyes followed her gaze, and he saw Ali. His blue eyes became cold, and he turned away with Celia. They skied off smoothly. They look like the perfect couple, thought Ursula bitterly.

****

Therapy Session

'OCD is characterized by persistent, intrusive, unwanted thoughts that the sufferer is unable to control. Such thoughts are often very distressing and result in discomfort. Many OCD sufferers also engage in rituals or compulsions that are persistent needs or urges to perform certain behaviour in order to reduce their anxiety or discomfort or to prevent some dreaded event from occurring. Most OCD sufferers can see the uselessness and absurdity of their actions but still feel compelled to perform their various rituals.'[3]

She seems to be performing origami with that map.

'Sorry Alexander, I was just trying to find the way to somewhere in Hampstead... Do you know if OCD causes you to have problems with finding your way to places? I'd be a dead loss as a homing pigeon.'
'I don't know. Undine, would you be able to give me the map?'
I stopped trying to fold the large square of recaltricant paper; my nerves tingled: 'Yes,' I handed it to Alexander quickly, in a flurry of colour, suddenly aware of my fingers touching it. He folded it easily and neatly and tucked it behind him on the chair.
'I have a couple of problem areas in my life,' I felt Ax focus. It's hard to concentrate when he looks deep into my eyes like this.
'A couple of problem areas...?'
'Oh, well, yes. I did wonder how much these rituals of touching things X number of times, are helping me to cope.'
'Good. And how well are the rituals helping?'
'They're not really. I need to make some progress, apart from anything else I'm running out of money. Since our last session, I thought that I would walk in today and say that I wanted to touch everything.'
'I wouldn't have asked you to do that, ever.'

'Well I want to touch things here now, not you,' I added
untruthfully. I still experienced the occasional urge to bonk
his socks off. They're dark green this session.
'Go ahead.'
'What?' I gaped at him.
'You said you wanted to touch things in this room, I said go
ahead.'

Alex watched as I took up my body and walked. I felt as
conspicuous as an agoraphobic and as articulated as a
marionette. Across to a side table, supporting a large ceramic
ashtray containing a set of keys. I carefully lifted the ashtray
and automatically looked for a manufacturer's stamp on the
base. I don't know why, as I wasn't interested, something to
make what I was doing appear normal. I could feel my fingers
already moving more than I wanted them to, across the
irregular glazed surface of the clay. There were no identifying
marks so I said lightly: 'Evening class pottery,' and set the
ashtray down clumsily. I turned towards the door and a
polished cabinet.
'Touch the surface of the cabinet,' Alex suggested.
I touched the smooth surface with four fingertips and felt my
heavy silver ring against the polished wood. Frightened, I
recoiled as though I'd been burnt and lurched back to my
seat.
'How do you feel?'
'Shell-shocked.'
'Anxiety-wise?'
'About three,' it didn't really seem a relevant measurement.
My knees began to shake, I was relieved to be sitting down.
'How likely do you think it is that you wrote something on any
of those things?'
'Not on the first, maybe on the second, I'm worse about the
third, maybe on the side or perhaps the underneath...'
'It's impossible for you to have done so.'
'That's not helping, it's not logical, the OCD.'
'No, I know.'
'I think the table is worse because you asked me to touch it, it
wasn't instigated by me.'
'And it's a flat surface.'
'Yes, maybe.'
'How are you going to deal with the need to check?'

'The hard thing is going to be not to check, when I leave.'
'How's your anxiety level now?'
'Getting worse about the table, whether I left words scratched on the side.'
That's what I do, escalate the anxiety myself.
''Getting worse' is no good Undine, I need numbers out of ten,' Alexander said impatiently. We'd had this discussion before.
'Seven!' I said coldly; it's very hard to equate numbers with emotional turmoil.

I said miserably: 'I can't ever use drawers or cupboards when staying somewhere, in case I leave marks or a piece of paper inside where I can't check easily. I can't put paper in envelopes without looking at it several times. I can't return Library books without flicking through all the pages and inspecting underneath the stamped label, again and again-'
'But we are going to work on this,' he interrupted. 'Using the Bank theory, that you have to have something in there in order to be able to withdraw it when needed.'
My Lloyds account is forever in deficit. I know there ain't enough self-compassion in me, unless something magical happens.
As though he was psychic, Alex said: 'You have to practice being compassionate towards yourself, that can be homework. We need to finish now.'
'But I often believe that I have written things in hidden places, like the underside of tables and chairs, and apart from scrabbling around under furniture, which I do sometimes, there's no way of checking. I suppose I could look at the underneath surface in a mirror and learn to read backwards. I'm the only person who goes to a friend's for a meal and doesn't touch the table once, all evening. It's so frustrating not being able to stop worrying about this!' I realised I was shouting, and stopped abruptly.
'I'm sure it is,' he said sympathetically, rising to show me out.

Undine

There's plenty of relaxed touching going on now.

....

I become aware that my right hand is resting laxly against the cool iron of the side of the wheelbarrow. My gaze lazily follows the wooden rafters across the underside of the sloping roof. Some drops of rain splatter onto the hut and against the tiny window. I can hear the wind musically stirring clattering foil bird-scarers strung across the next allotment. It's dry and warm in here, if rather crowded. Gabriel's leg straddles a pile of potatoes, bare foot resting half way up the wall. The earth moved at one point, off the scattered vegetables, most of it onto the floor. I look down tenderly at his golden head resting in the crook of my shoulder, a lock of his blonde hair trails across my breast. He seems to be sleeping; he has a beautiful skin.

****

The Therapist

His spermatozoa was like the rest of him – ambitious, devious and potent.
Trembling with shock in Tottenham Court Road opposite the turning to the hospital, Wendy shouted the news into her mobile 'phone above the din of traffic.
'I'm pregnant, they think it's twins.' After the call Alexander walked to the other end of the consulting room and stood at the window staring out at Eaton Place. Even insensitive Kelly, who had just arrived for Anger Management, realised something momentous was in the air. 'Was it bad news?' she asked hesitantly.
'What? Er...No'. Alexander remained with his back to her.
I could go,' she offered hopefully, 'I mean, we haven't started yet? I'm okay this week, I won't be mad at you.'
He turned with an effort, 'No, it's all right'. But he couldn't concentrate and did not see or hear much externally for the remainder of the sunny afternoon, the like of which he determined the twins should never live to see.

****

Undine

'Good luck, knock 'em dead!' That was Matilda. Chloris has lent me a smart wool skirt, so at least I look efficient. I've put drawings together in a sort of portfolio, including plans I drew up over the past fortnight of Einstein Road. These took ages, lots of the time spent enjoyably crawling beside skirting boards, measuring rooms with a dress-making tape measure. The sketches turned out surprisingly well, especially after I'd shaded them in. I also found some life drawings I did years ago at school and mounted them on card.

I was so worried about being late for the interview, that although it was only a couple of Tube stops away, I set off an hour beforehand, which meant I arrived at Bon Idee Designs twenty minutes early. It was housed in a modern building near the Heath. Marianne, the Receptionist was very friendly and gave me bottled water and made me a coffee as I sat nervously waiting. The room was lovely: light, and furnished in minimalist style with a glass and wood desk behind which Marianne was half-hidden, two Eames chairs, relaxing concealed lighting behind a narrow cornice running round the edge of the high ceiling, pale flawless carpet, a large vase of luxuriant flowers on a glass table and the hidden telephones purring with incoming calls. A couple of couriers were buzzed in, removing helmets with gloved hands, taking and delivering packages, joking with Marianne whilst signing the book. She smiled across at me: 'Marco's in a meeting Undine, he shouldn't be long. Would you like another coffee?'
'Oh no thanks, it's fine,' I said, dry-mouthed with nerves. Breathe Undine, in, one, two, three, four, five, six-seven-eightnineten, out, onetwothree-
'Good morning, Undine, thanks for being so punctual,' an Italian man, short and dark with a charming smile was advancing, holding out his hand.
'Okay Marianne, we'll be in Meeting Room one, no calls for half an hour please. I'll pick it up afterwards,' as Marianne held up a parcel.
'Good luck Undine,' she said, smiling. The 'phone rang: 'Good morning, Bon Idee Designs.'

I carefully picked up my case of drawings, and coat and followed Marco through silent swing doors, one of which he was holding open.

....

I had a wonderful evening in town with Gabriel. I told him all about the interview, I hope he wasn't bored. I liked Marco whom I'd be directly working to, and the other staff seemed equally friendly. It's a small company, only eight people, I really hope I get it. Marco thought my drawings showed talent, which did wonders for my ego. I can do something well which I really enjoy and might even get paid for, how wonderful is that? Interior Design-cum-Architecture seems rather a frivolous thing to do, but I can give money to charity once I've paid off my debts. The wages are quite good, there's training on the job and there's a chance of promotion eventually. I have to calm down, I haven't even been offered the job yet! Gabriel has got his fingers and metaphorical toes crossed for me.

We spent the evening wandering around the centre of town admiring architecture, eating a Thai meal – we didn't bother with any wine - finishing up with a coffee in Soho. Then I returned to Einstein Road on the last Tube. I feel clean and strong. Gabriel looked at me intently, half-smiling, before we kissed each other in Charing Cross Road, near Leicester Square tube. Very sexy. He texted me twice on the way home. He understands that I don't like talking on the 'phone, so SMSs are a perfect way of communicating. When he gave me the mobile phone, he said lightly it was because he didn't want to lose touch with me again.

****

Undine

I heard on the radio this morning that they want to genetically modify people. Scientists want to phase out flawed humans and create the 'perfect' species. I foresee protest marches by psychiatrists and psychotherapists, doctors, surgeons, nurses, criminologists … So Alex will be axed and redundant, a decorative dinosaur.

Alexander doesn't strike me as too much of a chameleon, because his mask is beginning to slip now I've known him a bit longer. He's coarsening and becoming sharper round the edges. It's the midnight of our relationship, I wonder what he'll turn into. He scowled when I arrived early this week and surprised him saying good-bye to a tall attractive woman, about his age. For some reason I don't think she's a patient. I heard him call her Wendy, I think it's the same person he told not to be tiresome, on the 'phone that time.

She was certainly in a state this time, angry and upset, standing outside at the top of the steps. Alexander was in the hall, his hand on the front door ready to close it, his expression haughtily irritable. That's when he looked past her and saw me. I looked up at Wendy sympathetically as I hesitantly mounted the steps, but she looked through me stonily, then averted her face as she hurried past me down to her car. It was almost as though she were jealous of me. She either had an awful cold or had been crying.

****

Therapy Session

<u>Anxiety Log</u>

	Mon.	Tues.	Wed.	Thurs.	Fri	Sat.	Sun.
Taps	5	5	6	5	0	3	4
Iron	6	6	5	6	0	4	5
Stove	7	4	5	4	0	4	4
Doors	4	5	4	5	0	2	2

'You and I have had a lot of interpersonal stuff going on between us,' Alex said gravely. I looked blank. Not as much as you obviously have with that tall, dark, estranged woman. Alex sounded as though he had a cold, but when I expressed sympathy he gave me an old-fashioned look and rapidly moved the subject away from himself. He explained what 'interpersonal' meant in terms of his work, but I couldn't really take it in. Apparently he has a new supervisor, but it was as though he was speaking through the glass wall again, and the glass stopped most of the meaning getting through.

Alex didn't notice on my Anxiety Log that I dealt with a flood, that was while I was staying at Helena's on Thursday night, and recorded zeros for the day afterwards. I was going to talk to him about Gabriel, but Alex was so brusque and focused on us practicing exposure to taps, that I didn't have an opportunity. The exposure work entailed me trotting in and out of the bathroom at the house again, turning taps on and off and touching mirrors, bath and basin, then not checking afterwards. This was far more demanding than it sounds, plus he had me touching doors and walls in the hall and not checking afterwards. He watched the build-up of tension in my face, monitoring how well I was coping, which before Gabriel I'd have utilised on the fantasy front. Alexander was supportive, standing next to me in the hallway and sweeping his hands across the plaster, touching the large ornate doors. This made my rituals appear so ludicrous and embarrassing that I didn't know whether to laugh or cry, so eventually did both. He briefly massaged my shoulders when I froze with tension. Prior to meeting Gabriel again I'd have found this overwhelming, let alone the aversion therapy. As it was, I think I looked fairly normal as his warm hands closed over the tops of my arms (well as sane as you can look when you are terrified of touching a door) but I'm still far from indifferent to Alexander.

After a while, he left me touching the inside of the front door. When I couldn't stand it any longer, I was beginning to feel faint, I timidly re-entered the consulting room to see him hurriedly writing up another patient's notes. I know this because at first I thought it was mine, but after a couple of minutes Alexander got up and dropped the file on to the desk next to me. My folder was upright on his chair, slightly bent: he'd been sitting against it. There were a couple of patients' files open on the desk, easily readable, but I turned away from them in my chair. I'm worried now that other people will be able to read mine.

I hate being a patient! I had a drink with Helena later, she works at an alcohol and drugs dependency unit, and she said nomenclature didn't matter: 'clients' or 'patients' equals the same thing. Alexander refers to his 'colleagues' constantly, which makes me feel a pariah, exiled out in the cold, a person who is not part of the 'norm'. Reminiscent of being in the bosom of my loving family, in fact. Once or twice, Alexander has let slip surprisingly patronising comments about patients, particularly in view of the fact he's talking to me. He objects to rudeness in his clients, but is intrinsically discourteous himself. If he and his colleagues find patients such a nuisance, why are they doing the job? If there is a Them and Us, we are the people who pay their wages. Perhaps all us weirdos should unite and stop using private therapists, that would send them mad.

I loathe being discussed by Alex with his supervisor, being defined as a case. I loathe it so much I don't know what to do with myself. I want to get out of this body, this brain. It's like when I first hated Grania. I didn't know any rude words except 'bum', being about four, so I sat on the bed in my chilly room, saying it over and over again. Black hate. I remember standing on tiptoe trying to slam the kitchen door, I couldn't reach the handle properly but made it bang anyway. My step-mother chased me furiously along the hall, I don't remember if she hit me. I just remember sitting on the bed staring furiously at nothing.

The reason I'm sounding off in this disillusioned and furious fashion is that the love bubble is deflating fast. So fast I can hardly breathe. I can't believe I've colluded with Alexander's unsavory attitude, by not tackling him on how irresponsibly he behaves in a position of trust. Instead of which I've kept quiet, not wanted to be a nuisance, even tried to save his feelings. The man doesn't have any! Face up to another unsavory fact Undine, you did it from lust.

....

Oh, these feelings for Alexander! Right, let's work through this and see if I can heal myself.
What if I told him how I felt, and he reached across and touched me gently, watching me. Well, that would be that, Utter Heaven. Wow! How likely is that to happen? Zero.

What if he listened, then said, 'So you really want to have sex with me Undine?'
'Oh yes!' (Croak.)
'Come on then,' peeling off his clothes in the middle of the consulting room.
'Stop, I can't, I mean you can't - it's supposed to be a professional relationship -' (Provided I wasn't so mesmerised by the emerging torso that I couldn't speak.)
'Well make up your mind!'
Alexander putting his trousers back on in a huff.

What if we didn't click in bed?

Better kept as fantasy then: otherwise tons more grief and embarrassment to ruminate over in the small hours, and the inconvenience of having to find a new therapist.

****

Torquil

I was woken by loud scraping noises from above, I thought Gabriel had gone to work, perhaps I dreamed it. I didn't get in until five this morning. Chris and I went Clubbing, then he had to be up for a breakfast meeting so I came home so as to avoid being woken early. What time is it? Ten-thirty... Want a slash anyway. What if it isn't Gabriel? A burglar? I pulled on my robe: 'Gabriel,' I called, my voice sounded rather shaky. The scraping stopped. Then I could hear footsteps going into the kitchen and water running away down the pipes. I trod into my slippers, and shivering - when will he put a stove down here too? – went to the bottom of the ladder. I could see up into the hall above; whoever it was continued to clatter things together in the kitchen. My heart was thumping.

I climbed up the iron ladder, then as my head emerged at floor level, the door to the hall suddenly clicked open. I nearly fell off my perch with fright - so did she. A girl was standing there holding a bucket and mop, wearing a sweater and jeans. That's Gabriel's jumper!

'Who are you?' we both demanded in unison. 'I'm Undine ... Are you Torquil?' she asked, relaxing slightly.

'Yes.' So this is Cat-Woman! Posh voice, blonde, skinny, pretty I suppose - in an anaemic sort of way.

'I didn't know you were in Torquil, sorry. I hope I didn't wake you?' she said nicely.

'I thought you were a burglar! Pleased to meet you,' I reached the hall floor and smiled kindly at her. 'Okay if I have a shower?' I opened the bathroom door.

'Oh yes, of course,' Undine backed away with her bucket, and disappeared into the sitting-room, quietly closing the door.

After my ablutions, I went into the sitting-room and stopped dead with shock. The front door was propped open with a chair, outside a bright, cold, sunny morning beckoned. I could see the ducks on the pebbles, a tiny bird was bobbing around pecking at the mud. It was low tide. The table was on the deck, the sofa was pulled into the centre of the room, the blinds had been taken down. I walked through into the kitchen:

'What's going on?' My voice came out sounding strange. There's nothing wrong with my cleaning! The room wavered through a mist of anger.

'I just thought I'd give it an early spring-clean for Gabriel, the blinds were really dirty, I hosed them down outside and I'll finish them off in the bath later. I found all sorts of things behind the sofa.' She wrinkled her nose.

I maintained a haughty silence and pointedly took a plate from the drying rack.

'Oh sorry, I expect you want breakfast. There's some coffee still hot in the cafetiere if you'd like some Torquil, and some bagels in the bread bin.' She beamed at me.

That bitch's telling me what I can and can't do, in my home! A baaygel! I want some scrambled eggs! Where's that nice saucepan? Not on its hook... Oh here, in the new sink, soaking! How anal, she's even got those black marks off, I thought they were burnt on. I can't find my wooden spatula. I began rifling noisily through drawers. 'Have you seen my wooden spatula?' I asked with frigid politeness, poking my head round the doorway to the sitting-room.

'No, I don't think so,' she said, looking unconcerned.

As I banged around crossly in the kitchen, Undine switched on the Hoover. In the end, I just grabbed my bag without having any breakfast and stormed out. The effect was a bit wasted as she was scrubbing something in the bathroom and I couldn't move the chair sufficiently out of the way to slam the front door. As I leapt off the beer crates I saw my spatula. It was outside in the firewood box.

****

Undine

I've been antagonistically reacting to Alexander as a person, as a diversionary tactic to avoid scaling the emptiness inside myself to find the true, but still weak, muscle of Self. Vertiginous on an epic scale, in fact. [Has there been any substance to this text yet?]. La!

But Alex is not doing performing his job the way this book says he should be. When I told Matilda this she said, that's probably why he didn't want you to read about OCD. It doesn't mean he's not good at his work. If you sail in there and start telling him how to do his job, it'll drive such a wedge between you the treatment won't work anyway.

No wonder Alex didn't want to me to read this stuff: it's so reassuring. Well, apart from the sentence: 'Repeatedly employing prolonged exposure (45 minutes to 2 hours) to the obsessional cues with strict response prevention allows habituation to take place'.[*]
Can't see myself ever being able to achieve that without clones arriving in Armani coats to whip me off for incarceration. The rest of the chunk I read though, about 20 pages, constantly reiterated doing things at the patient's own pace, being sensitive and aware. It was also couched in easily accessible language. Of course, this is the first medical text I've dared peruse, but considering I felt as though a black mamba might drop from between the leaves, I emerged light-headed with relief. I also feel fractionally more in control.

Which meant I began reading other medical books and most of them seemed to be on similar lines: Foa et al[*] posit that the younger the individual when symptoms of OCD began, the better the improvement was maintained at follow-up. Good, I can remember carefully filling my pockets with cigarette ends at five years old, so that the village wouldn't burn down. Apparently a number of reports suggest that a combined approach of behavioural therapy and medication is the most favoured, but this is briskly shot down by someone else who states that there is little evidence to support this recommendation for the majority of sufferers. Think I'll stick to doing without medication for as long as I can.

I do feel a chill when I read that I have an 'illness', I'm uneasy at being labelled mentally ill, it makes me feel incapable of making fair, 'normal' or truthful choices. Even words are failing me here. Just as I was beginning to feel able to make decisions, without turning myself inside out as to whether I was being fair. Before I come across as some kind of Saint, this scrupulousness only comes into play towards people I dislike, or feel intimidated by.

One paragraph made me laugh aloud: before you say anything, I'm one of the afflicted so I can laugh at anything to do with OCD. They discovered that patients who believed their fears were realistic and that their behavioural rituals might well prevent an actual disaster from occurring, tended not to benefit from exposure treatment. Well, what a surprise! I rescind my theory that genius is stating the unstated self-evident.

Alexander knows both more and less than I thought, which makes me respect him a bit more again. What a weird way to make your living though.

****

Undine

Alex is transmitting his peculiar aura of calm and charm again. Not enough to get me to divulge stuff about my brother, but I prattle on fairly easily.
'Don't let me hi-jack the session will you?' I ask him at one point. 'I mean, you must have a system.'
'I think these issues are relevant. I hadn't realised that your mother died when you were so young.' I was sure I'd told him once before, but didn't say anything.

I care more about people in the abstract, than I do about people supposedly close to me. I ask Alex if that makes me a psychopath. It's the end of a session so he's doing that metamorphosing-into-a-distant-castle thing he sometimes does. It means he's focused on being in a hurry to get somewhere or do something without sacrificing courtesy, but only just. Silence as Ax puts things in his bag with his back to me, 'No, I don't think you are,' he says eventually as though from a long way away.
'Are you sure?' I can't help the need for reassurance, panic is on the up.
But that's all I'm going to get. He's as hard as flint, almost frightening, if I transgress the boundaries of what's good form and permissible. I can just manage, through employing good old back-boned courtesy myself, to leave with my ego intact.

****

Person with depression: 'No one spoke to me all evening.'
What, no-one?'
'No, no-one.'
'Not even the waitress?'
'Well, yes, but she only asked me if I'd like a drink.'

I've just read about someone with depression, feeling
miserable after an evening of believing themselves ignored.
There's that supposed link sometimes between depression
and OCD – scarcely surprising – so I'm reading up a bit about
feeling low. Decided I may have a prosperous future at some
point, as I'm already an expert on the condition. I can relate to
the unfortunate person having problems socialising, because
up until a couple of years ago I used to go home in a haze of
misery after a night out, reliving all the embarrassing things I'd
said, who'd ignored me or said something hurtful, etcetera -
Da de da, as Annie Hall would say.

But I do have irrepressible visions of the person, above,
standing facing the wall, drink in hand, while people tap them
on the shoulder and try in vain to talk to them. I'm jealous, as
my hang-up is compulsive chattering. I've just thought: if it's a
her and she's aged 40 plus, I've heard women of that age
commenting that they suddenly seem to have become
invisible. Women can't win; when too young emotionally to
cope with all the unwanted sexual attention, girls are suddenly
under a spotlight. I'm speaking from experience here, so just
bear me out.

Just as women have learned how to deal with being a minor
celebrity, apparently the spotlight suddenly moves on, leaving
them stranded on a dark stage. Something to look forward to
then, along with the menopause. Before you say this is a
blessing regarding unwanted lecherous attentions from
strangers, that bit doesn't always apply either. Helena's mum
assured me that there will be still be some pot-bellied, leering,
smelly, cerebrally-challenged individual who's never doubted
their own attraction (invariably male), who can still see you.
They make plumbing noises whilst sidling around within your

personal space, fingers like tentacles. Meanwhile apparently attractive and intelligent people suddenly start repeating what you've just said as their idea, barge into you on the pavement - particularly if you're struggling along with heavy supermarket bags – stop asking what you do at parties, insist they were ahead of you in a queue and attempt to run you over in their cars. This all with the glad cry of: 'Oh, I didn't see you!' So I'll suggest to Alex he check out the age, if the patient is female. Chances are they're not depressed at all, just murderously pissed off.

****

Undine

I was offered the job as Assistant Interior Designer! I'm ecstatic and everyone has been really sweet. Gabriel bought me some Rotring pens; Matilda, Dion, Chloris, Helena, Finn and some other friends came out to celebrate at the Hawley Arms, after which we had fish and chips at Lisson Grove. They all seemed to like Gabriel, especially Matilda and Helena who find him extremely attractive, although Matilda didn't phrase it that delicately.

I've been working in my new job for a month now, and everything's going smoothly. Everyone's very busy but helpful and I'm learning all the time, which means I'm exhausted in the evenings, but very happy. I'm in danger of becoming conceited. I've already arranged to hold an exhibition of my drawings in March next year, at an artist's studios called the 'Pavillion', near *The Ark*. Gabriel showed me the venue a couple of months ago when we first walked to the Farmer's Market at Duke's Meadows to buy organic bread. Marianne saw one of the flyers on my desk and everyone at work has kindly said they'll come to the exhibition. It's a bit daunting, but I'm getting quite a lot of painting done on the boat at week-ends. In fact it'll coincide with the Bon Idee Annual Outing (or 'grand piss-up' as Marianne terms it) so they're considering a river cruise afterwards.

The only fly in the ointment is Torquil, I'm not sure if he likes me. Gabriel says he does, but Torquil seems to avoid me, and says ambiguous things when our paths do cross. I don't want to spoil their friendship, but Gabriel says everything's fine.

****

Undine

Alexander had rung me, ostensibly to arrange the next session: I'd already admitted I was having a bit of a panic attack. He said: 'You're human. So long as you don't attach more to it,' which I didn't understand.
'Um, I know I've probably asked you this before Undine, but your file is locked away in the other office. What is your history of medication?'
'None.' I said proudly and rather indignantly. How come he didn't remember that?
'Ah. Why is that?' He was eating something, chewing loudly.
'I feel as though you want me to take medication.'
No, I was just wondering. It's just that you said you were going to read those books about OCD and I am concerned about what you'll read in them. There can be a lot about drugs, and pathopsychological medicine ...'
'I've read that the combination of drugs and OCD is supposed to be the best way, though I haven't read much yet ...'
He swallowed liquid with a loud gulp: 'Some people are upset by the idea of taking medication, but others are perfectly happy to try something.'
'I don't like taking medicine that's "good" for me, unless I absolutely have to.' I've 'self-medicated' with way too much alcohol in the past, but he should remember that.
'The thing is, the format in some of these books relates to two hours of exposure techniques.'
I laughed. 'I couldn't handle that.'
'I know, you and some others would have left. If you had to write something resting on a table say, then not look at it or the table for two hours.' Alexander was talking with his mouth full, surprisingly uncouth for him. 'You're responding quite well to treatment, as we take it gently.'

'I'm a bit worried now, that I'm not progressing as fast as other patients because we take it slowly.'
'That's an interesting way of looking at it.'
'It's because I'm very competitive.'
'As I've said to you before, my concern is that we've been having too long and too many breaks between sessions. It felt much better this week because I didn't have to remember where we had got up to, and we didn't have to...' (pause while he thinks how best to phrase it, but I know what he's going to say) '... get past your reluctance to talk about it again.'

I wished he'd stop masticating in my ear.

'It did feel more relaxed this week. I know why I've never taken medication, it's because my step-mother's been on tablets since I was little.'
'Yes, I remember you not wanting medication now. The first time I asked, you said: "Why, do you think I'm mad?"'
I laughed. 'I don't actually think being mad is bad, it's interesting. It's just a shame it always seems to be such an unhappy state. Do you think I need medication?'
'No.'
'I'm going to be reading more of those books for research purposes, I want to try writing some articles for newspapers. Can I have a debriefing session after going through the books?' I found I was laughing again, purely a social mechanism.
'Yes, but if you get very frightened during the next two weeks while I'm on holiday, you can ring me for a ten-minute chat.'
'Are you sure?'
'Yes. If it's really necessary.' He belched.

I checked that Alex had definitely rung off in case I rang off abruptly and then felt terrible. From my breezy 'phone manner, I fell abruptly into tears. I felt utterly inadequate and he obviously had me down as a complete scaredy-cat, just when I'd begun believing I was quite brave after all. So ended a caring, but misjudged 'phone call from him. Alexander probably only rang me to make himself feel better before he went on yet another holiday, I thought uncharitably.

****

Torquil

"All the suicides wash up round Hammersmith Bridge, something to do with the currents."
I can't look where the Rupert the Instructor is pointing as I'm feverishly trying to row in time with Number One oar. It's like learning to swim: the harder you try the more difficult it is. Number One's blade lifts fast and clean from the brown water, silver droplets sparkling along the blade, before turning again to enter the Thames. Bet he's not really a beginner – very boyish though, with gorgeous black hair, so glossy it gleams silver in the Autumn sunlight.

I can't lust after Gareth for long; my soaked trainers are wedged beneath leather straps, that I pull against to propel my wooden seat on castors back and forth in time with the strokes. My bum's numb. I can't invite him casually to the pub afterwards because I'm sitting in a pool of water and will look like an advert for failed incontinence breeches. It's disconcerting not knowing where you're going - shooting along jerkily backwards as we are. What happens if we capsize? Will I be able to undo the foot straps before drowning upside-down? Perhaps we'll be outside *The Ark* by then and Gabriel will act as Noah! He could save me *and* Gareth and take us aboard as an endangered species. Actually he'd probably let us drown at the moment, *if* he even noticed us drifting past, he's so besotted with Airhead Undine.

But I'm lucky compared to Sheila; she only went rowing once because her oar got trapped painfully under her ample bosom as she was ricocheting forward on the little hard trolley. Apparently the boat ploughed to a halt, despite the other seven crew members manfully trying to row onwards. Better than a Wonderbra. I'd rather drown than asphyxiate head-first in my own cleavage.

"Right" shouts the Cox suddenly, standing up beefily in the stern: "Oars should be just above the water, then we can balance, can't we? Otherwise," he rocks ferociously from side to side "the boat becomes low in the water." Sweat rolls

down my stomach, making my white vest even wetter and now there's mud on my shorts, despite my efforts to look my best in case Gareth turned up a second week running. That little bully is still over-compensating by shouting.
"Come forward to row. What was that Number Three? It's a very safe sport, don't be a big girl's blouse. You can swim, can't you? Now, when I say ready, *when* I say it, GO!"

I used to avoid rowing because of those bossy girls sporting Wellingtons and post-skiing suntans outside river-side pubs. They carry their oars, even into the toilets, and yell things like "Wasn't Jeremy great at Henley, Caz?" It never occurred to me that the boys would be just as crass.

The first time I went out on the river, last week, it went really well. The wooden boat, the swirling current, sporadic evening sunlight emerging from clouds to illuminate crisp packets floating upstream. Then Acne Henry in our boat lost the beat and the oar handle shot up and smacked his teeth together like one of those old-fashioned nutcrackers. I expect his girlfriend's been wanting to do that for ages when he loses the rhythm. I wondered patronisingly why he found rowing so difficult.

This week I'm the prat in the boat and just want to go home. My new vest is now a muddy ruin due to other Beginners catching crabs.
Okay nurse, I admit it, I caught them on Wednesday evening in a boat with several fit oarsmen near Putney -
"Concentrate Number Three. Yes, you! And for God's sake *try* and stop hitting Gareth there in the back!" I jumped nervously, lost the rhythm and kneed Gareth hard in the kidneys.
"Tosser!" he roared.
"Sorry," I muttered, burning with embarrassment. Gareth craned round to give me an evil look. His eyes were unattractively blood-shot.

At this point another crew flew past us quietly on the River Styx with a synchronised hiss, their oars effortlessly pushing the water away. The bronzed rowers were sleekly decked out in Lycra emblazoned with Club colours, revealing be-muscled thighs. I wonder where those guys hang out?

****

Therapy Session

I was ten minutes early. Filling in time, I walked past the mansion block on the opposite side of the street, glancing at the windows and wondering who was in the hot seat. It was windy, the sky pewter behind the buildings and trees. The weather glancing from light showers and rainbows to darkness and back to bright cold sunlight again. Just before I rounded the corner at the end of the road, I looked back, and saw a movement inside the large porch of Alex's building. Marius suddenly materialised at the top of the steps. I stopped dead. He leapt down the stairs two at a time and ran away from me towards the Tube station. He had been pushing something glittering and metallic inside his unzipped jacket with his right hand. I looked at my watch, it was time for my appointment. I tried to breathe deeply, but panic closed my throat. I rang the bell, wondering if I was leaving marks on it, and climbed back down a step so as not to be too close to Alex when he answered the door. If he answered it.

Alex seemed unharmed, he was peering into my folder. 'I'm sorry Alexander,' I said breathlessly, as I sat in my usual seat (his, since the time I'd complained of feeling uncomfortable in my allotted seat and we'd swapped).
'I had the most awful panic attack, just now.' I had to say something to excuse my frantic state. My stomach lurched as I stared round the expensively-appointed room. What if Marius had done something awful here or broken something? I felt cold dread.
'Oh that's interesting, I wanted to work with you on something connected with that.'
With Marius? No, no, Alex was talking about panic. With difficulty I switched my gaze to him. He opened his pad: 'Let me just write this out.'
As he wrote, I tried to breathe deeply in the soothing silence, endeavouring to reason. I must ring Chloris. Alex finished writing a couple of minutes later and leaned back and crossed

his legs. He surveyed me calmly, pushing his hair back with a casual hand.

'How did you feel on the way here?'

'Awful, I told you.' Marius wasn't usually jealous, but he had changed at the end of our relationship.

'At the risk of sounding pedantic, it's probably best not to term it 'awful'. If it was a total panic attack, what do you think would have happened?'

'I wouldn't have got here?'

'That's right'

'But it was terrible, sweats, shakes and dreads.'

'Okay, call it very difficult, horrible, but not 'awful' Undine. I'm managing to look at Alexander without feeling dazzled. Probably because I'm irritated by this bewildering insistence on semantics. Doubtless enlightenment will dawn later. I'll only be here for an hour, then I can call Matilda, I think I can remember her mobile number if she's not at home, and see if she's got Chloris' work number.

I remembered something and interrupted Alexander – I hadn't heard what he'd been saying:

'I'm sorry, I have to tell you while I remember- I'm not bothering to fill in an Anxiety Log any more as it's stayed the same for three weeks. Most things at 5 or 6 or less.'

'Okay,' he said slowly. 'But you need to start filling it out again soon because it will change and you'll be able to monitor your progress.'

'All right,' I agreed reluctantly. I hate having to think about my OCD behaviour all the time, it's tiring. Plus it's a drag having to make notes, although I don't panic so much now about using a pen.

'Alexander…'

'Yes,'

'Um- What do you do if a patient becomes too keen on you, I mean have you ever had anyone stalk you?'

'No,' he looked at me, surprised. 'Well, not that I know of …Why?' he smiled politely.

I felt renewed dread. 'Well, what would you do if a patient became too fond of you, say, and then their partner got angry?'

He now looked perplexed and concerned. 'I'd refer the patient to a colleague of mine,' he said slowly.

'It's all right, it's just that I'm thinking of writing a story about something like that,' I lied hurriedly.

'Did you feel like running away when you had the panic attack?'

'I don't allow myself to think like that, but coming to see you is akin to visiting the dentist. Nothing personal.' Most of this was true, I had had panic attacks of course, but without the complication of catching Marius behaving strangely.

'What were you worried about?'

'Nothing to do with the session, I felt pleased earlier this morning, because I was coming to see you. Then it swung round, it began while I was waiting for the Tube train. I know it's not you, it's to do with me.'

He nodded approvingly. 'What happened?'

'I don't know, I just began to feel scared.'

'What were you frightened of?'

The unknown. 'Um, what might come up during the session.'

'Ah,' his pen scratched on the smooth paper, resting on my folder on his knees.

I warmed to my minor fear: 'I'm not going to be able to cope afterwards.'

He wrote busily. 'I'm just doing this so that we can work with it in a minute. How are you feeling?'

'Fine now.'

'You were concerned about what was going to come up during the session, and that you wouldn't be able to cope afterwards. Was there anything else you thought?'

'And that it won't be contained in the session, which is down to you.' This sounded aggressive, but it felt too late to rephrase it.

'....contained in the session.' He wrote at the top of the page. Alex read aloud what he'd written. My thoughts became vague with incomprehension. 'Sorry, it feels like my listening problem, anxiety with the 'phone? Could I read it?'

'Of course,' he proffered the sheet. 'Read it aloud to me though.'

'How did you know I was going to have a panic attack on the way here? You said you wanted to work with me a certain way.'

'I didn't, but it's useful. This is ABC.'

Acronyms! CBT, ABC... Hope it doesn't go up to Z or I'll be here until I die.

'I apologise if I smell of smoke, I've just had a cigarette.'
'You don't,' I said automatically, before realizing that Alex was
moving closer to show me the sheet. His shirt sleeve brushed
my arm. He didn't smell of smoke, he smelt faintly and
deliciously of expensive soap. I hurriedly read aloud:

'A: Going to Alex's
  What's going to come up?

B: I'm not going to be able to cope afterwards.
  It won't be contained in the session.'

C: Anxiety and Avoidance Behaviour.'

'Is it realistic to say: "I'm not going to be able to manage after
the session?"' Alex asked.
'I haven't always managed well...'
'All right, but how often in relation to the times you have
coped?'
'Less times.'
'Is it constructive to say it?'
'No.'
'Why not?'
'It becomes a self-fulfilling prophecy?'
And of course, finally, ' He pointed to the third word in the list
at the top of the page.
'Compassionate. It could be compassionate to realise that
I'm not going necessarily to manage well,' I argued.
'But if you imagine someone saying to you:' You're not going
to manage well,' that's not believing in your abilities, or
acknowledging that you've coped well in the past.'
'True.'
Let's find a different way of saying things; how could you say
'I'm not going to be able to cope afterwards' in a gentler way?'
'Sometimes I've had difficulty coping afterwards and I'm
worried about that this time?'
'Good, can you add to that?'
I can't think. Alex reads out words to me again, doesn't he
remember that that doesn't always work? I can't concentrate.
I remember a sunny classroom at the village primary school,
high old-fashioned windows, and smirking as I was told to
count brightly-coloured buttons at the front of the sums class

as a ritual of humiliation, I must have been eight. Mrs Flame was known for being strict, and had a wart on her face and grey permed hair, but I didn't dislike her. When I was five I had a different, slightly less fearsome, teacher as I tried to learn how to read the word 'said'. I had problems with that too, but only for a short time.

'It's all right, you don't have to give the right answer,' he said now, smiling at me.
I sagged with relief. 'I feel as though I should,'
'What's this 'should'? It's like "ought", "must", "will", "have to". There's no "should" - words like that put an unreasonable demand on people.'
'I'm scared of appearing thick. I always used to pretend I understood when people were telling me things, which confused them and landed me in trouble.'
'Yes, that's anxiety blocking understanding, it happens to everyone when they're anxious.' This was reassuring.
'But we've done this before haven't we?
'Just because we did this once several sessions ago, and have just had a long break, why should you remember it Undine? Please read out the first part again,' he gave me the sheet and folder to hold.
'Sometimes I've had difficulty coping afterwards and I'm worried about that this time… I could add that I'll talk to Alex about it when I get to the session?'
I don't feel that it is all right to telephone Alex between sessions, despite being encouraged to, having heard him speak disparagingly of other patients' calls.
'Yes,' he wrote busily.
How does this look?' He handed me another sheet, 'Can you read my scrawl?'
'Yes,' I began reading aloud but paused half-way through because I was self-conscious about my voice. 'Sorry, but at the school I attended, they used to take the micky, saying that I talked 'posh', so I accommodated. Now I've lost a lot of my vocabulary and speak lazily.'
'Probably a desire to be liked.'
'But some people always picked up something, however hard I tried.'

'They would. I think it's about sharing one's humanity, ultimately. All you can do is your best, that goes for everyone - we are all only human.'
'Yes.' I agreed totally, but silently wondered if one can surmount other people's prejudice.

Eureka! The key is in how you view other people. If you're feeling afraid that if you look up, that there is a wall of judgmental eyes critically watching your every move, then you are going to start carrying out safety procedures in, for example, the supermarket. In my case, that means nerving myself to pick up a bottle of washing up liquid, hopefully it's the ecological type, but if I inadvertently pluck Phosphate Concentrate from the shelf I'm incapable of putting it back because I've touched it. After I've dropped it gingerly into my basket, I then stand on tiptoe to inspect the shelf space from whence it came to see whether I've touched a bottle nearby, or loosened a cap, or left a mark on the shelf, blah blah blah. Because I'm behaving so furtively, I become a magnet for unimaginative store detectives: sturdy women with sensible shoes, and men with no necks. So you see why shopping for necessities can take some time and why I don't always return home with the right products. So much for free choice.
Alex was speaking.
'Sorry?'
'We have to finish now, do you have any questions Undine?'
'Why's it not all right to use 'awful'?'
Alex explained that certain words affect the consciousness in a particular way.

It occurred to me that there might be a problem defining what different words mean to different people. Professional pedanticism must be awkward to implement when Alexander of the Aristocratic Voice, meets East End gangster:
'I'm gutted Al,'
'Could you define 'gutted' for me Jason?'
'Uh?'
'Perhaps we could substitute 'a bit upset', what do you think?'
'You taking the piss or what?'
[*Violent noises off.*]

****

I rang Chloris, but her 'phone was engaged. I hurried home and told Matilda in full how I'd seen Marius. We discussed it for ages but decided early on not to call the police, as nothing seemed to have happened. Chloris came in, both she and Matilda denied having told Marius anything about Alexander. Matilda said: 'Do you think Marius stole something? You said it was silvery, whatever he was hiding in his jacket.'
I couldn't remember seeing anything silver in the hall or consulting room, but that didn't mean much, the house was enormous.
'It could have been a knife, or something to get into the building with, said Chloris, worried.
'Marius has got a knife!'
Chloris and Matilda looked horrified. 'I'm going to have to tell Alexander,' I said reluctantly. 'He might be at risk.'

....

I 'phoned Alexander with my usual trepidation; I could visualise his thick sleek hair and warm face against the receiver at the other end. Listening to the repetitive ringing tone, I worried about what would happen if I said something provocative.
Stop OCD-ing, Undine.
'Yes,' it was a woman's voice. I was bewildered: perhaps I had the wrong number.
'Is - is Alexander there?'
'No. Who is this?' She sounded cold and haughty. Panic wiped my brain, I momentarily forgot my own name.
'Um, er – I'll call him back … later.'
The receiver was slammed down at the other end.

****

Marius

Bloody hell, Swizz's workplace was posh. Exclusive area, massive Victorian consulting room, all fancy plasterwork, good stuff, and bits of art - not so good by a long chalk - dotted carefully around on antique, gleaming furniture. Why should he have all this, and me bugger-all? In a moment of

rage, I grabbed this baby's head, life-size – it seemed very light for terracotta - and hurled it with all my strength at the wall, expecting it to shatter. It bounced off and landed with a thud on a plush Chinese rug where it rolled. I couldn't believe it. When I picked it up to look, it was made of plastic and cardboard, not what it seemed at all. I dropped it into a fancy waste bin. Suddenly I heard footsteps in the corridor, I grabbed a silver paper knife off the desk. But then I heard voices approaching; I didn't want to meet the bastard with someone else as witness. Quickly I slipped through a doorway at the end of the room, at the same moment the main door opened. I'd clocked the two exits when I arrived. I softly padded across the hall towards some steps that I guessed led down to the basement. I glanced up just before the bend in the staircase, to see the back of a guy with coiffed dark hair and an expensive leather jacket. He was droning on in a toff's voice: it sounded familiar, not from the 'phone I mean, and something about the way he was standing … I remember people. It was Alex Stinger! Mind you 'Swizz' will do just as well. We overlapped briefly doing time. A very classy conman. I'm surprised they caught him, the other cons used to refer to him as Teflon Man behind his back, but Stinger got greedy. Now as Alex slowly pushed the door closed behind him I took a big risk, shot up the steps, slid along the hall and out of the front door. I'm not mixing it with him, he's put people in hospital. Fucking hell - maybe it was him who cracked me over the head at Undine's!
Just found myself in a bloody bush outside Einstein Road, with a splitting headache and birds tweeting in a circle. All the more reason for lying low, plenty more fish in the sea. Undine was too much like hard work anyway.

****

Alexander

'I didn't get where I am today by not putting demands on myself!' Echoes of Reggie's boss in the *The Rise and Fall of Reginald Perrin*.
'You're in a Shrink's chair.' I reminded the middle-aged, plump guy who was wearing expensive corduroys, and Church's brogues. He'd draped his rain-soaked Aquascutum

over the back of his seat and it was dripping on the floor. I began to worry that it would ruin Harry's latest exotic rug, he's always adding things to the consulting-room.
'Oh. Yes.'
Sean Barham is beginning to get on my nerves, I look discreetly at my watch, twenty minutes left.
'Let me just hang this in the hall for you, it might dry quicker near the radiator.' I reverently removed the mackintosh from his chair.
Doesn't matter that Sean Barham has earned himself £8 million and made £20m for his firm, he'll always be unhappy until he gets past having had a disapproving bully for a father. Which is money in the Bank.

Oh for f---- sake! David's absent-mindedly taken the keys to the filing cabinet home with him again. I'm going to have to wing it with the next appointment. The only thing I can remember about Undine, apart from her name (at least I've got that off now), is that hurtful remark she made about me being more charm than compassion. I've done a lot of kind things in my time.

****

PRESENT

I've just had this awful evening session with Alexander, I don't know how to manage. I gradually realise that I'm on the 'Westbound' platform at the Tube station, instead of returning across town to Einstein Road. So, Gabriel then. I don't have the energy to struggle up steps against the flow of strangers, to change platforms. When I disembark in a daze at Turnham Green, an E3 bus screeches to a halt at the stop beside me, it seems fated. It'll deposit me only yards from *The Ark*.

It's November, not long until the longest night now. I sit there, a frozen alien, in the bus. It seems warm, bright and full, I'm surrounded by people carrying Christmas shopping, some chatting animatedly and two excited small children holding onto a pushchair containing a full Hamleys carrier bag, parked in the space near the back doors. Eventually though, there is only me and an old red-faced benevolent drunk left. Then there's just me walking like an automaton towards the river, seeing my breath blooming white in the dark-blue frosty air. I look down at the deck of *The Ark* before I open the gate to the ramp – to see the outside light on and Sheila standing very close to Gabriel. He says something and she laughs, he is smiling. Suddenly she puts her arms around him and her mouth to his, running her fingers through his hair. It all seems to happen so fast and then to last for a long time. I can't believe what I'm seeing. I can't bear seeing it. The dazzling deck light shimmers. I turn and after a while realise that I'm stumbling, as if drunk, back along the bank towards Hammersmith.

....

She's been lost, meaning to go to Hammersmith Tube station, but wandering haphazardly across busy roads leading to the huge roundabout, without ever homing in on the station and familiarity and safety. Eventually she realises that the Odeon is on her left beneath the ugly roaring flyover, with *The Ark* office building containing vacant, brightly-lit rooms above and behind her. The Church rises dimly further along on the left, the clock striking eleven, with a stretch of grass in front and the cross, dark and dwarfed by the high frontage housing the shops and Tube station, it's reflection shimmering palely upon the glass towering wall of offices. She leaves it all behind, walking across Hammersmith Bridge; the panels shifting underfoot as a lone car passes. She passes beneath the long iron strips suspending the bridge in the air, massive nuts and bolts holding it in the ether. The unwieldy Victorian painted plaster porpoises gigantically posture at each end. She stops in the middle and looks over the edge at the a dim light on the side of the bridge, warning boat-owners of the massive brick piles pushing down into the silt. The gravity, depths and quietness of the deep river sliding beneath, awe her. The mud at the edges is still marginally visible, but the tide is coming in fast. A solitary rower skims beneath her on the deserted water, in a fragile skiff bearing a tiny light. 'Don't do it love, too cold,' says a woman shuffling past pulling a trolley, holding her dirty coat tightly to her throat.

....

Time passes. Frenzied thoughts return again and again, remembering and repeating her anxieties, interspersed with the final image of Gabriel kissing a woman with auburn hair. Suddenly her head is silent. She does not exist.
I want peace.
An intrusive voice, urgently loud: 'Undine?'
I seem to be coming back, reluctantly, from a long way away. 'Undine!'
The dark water swirls below again, I hear and see it closer now, gulping against the brick plinth. The iron parapet of the bridge is hard under my knees. The bridge reverberates with running footsteps. Gabriel appears a few feet away, looking at me, breathing fast. His face is drained of blood in the sodium light. Shocked, I stare back mutely, swaying back onto my heels. I'm freezing.
'Come on Undine, it's a bit chilly for hanging around on Hammersmith Bridge,' he says pleadingly, stopping and holding out his hands. I allow him to help me down from the parapet onto the pavement, then move away from him.
'I saw you kissing that woman,' I say eventually with a great effort. It doesn't appear relevant now, it was an age ago, but it seems important that it's said.

'I know, but it wasn't me kissing Sheila, it was her kissing me, I stopped it.'

We turn and walk silently across the deserted bridge onto land. Feeling is slowly returning, prickling pins and needles in my hands, they burn. I stop and push them into my armpits to try and stop the pain. Gabriel quickly removes his gloves and gently pulls them over my hands, they're wonderfully warm inside. He's looking down at me, he's still pale, he looks very concerned. 'Matthew mentioned that he'd seen you walking towards Hammersmith when I was getting rid of Sheila, so I ran after you. I couldn't find you!' I gradually realise that Gabriel has one arm loosely round my shoulders as we wander along the pavement slowly, his comforting warm body a shield between me and the darkness.
'But you did in the end,'
'Really because I asked this homeless woman and she remembered seeing you on the bridge, she was worried about you.'
'So kind,' I began to cry.
'Yes.' He stopped and wiped away my tears gently with his fingers. 'She wouldn't take any money.'
We stop: I realise we've reached the junction with the towpath. Gabriel's hair gleams fair in the moonlight.
'Would you like to stay on the boat tonight? I can sleep on the floor of the sitting-room if you like.'
'Yes... I don't know. The session tonight with the therapist before I saw you with Sheila ... Gabriel, it was awful.'
'Do you want to talk about it? I'm always here for you Undine.'
'Whatever I'd done?'
'Whatever you've done.'
'However bad it was,' I ask with a terrible effort, but the panic is overwhelming. 'If I'd murdered people, or things as bad or worse than that?' Let's get it over with. I stare up, Gabriel's eyes are dark hollows, he has his back to the streetlamp.
'Undine, I love you, I will always love you, however bad the things you've done are.' We start walking again. 'If you can put up with me, I'll never leave you. But I don't believe you've done evil things.'
I stop walking abruptly and turn to him.

'But I have! You're only saying you'll stay with me and everything because you don't really think I've done anything bad.'

'No darling, I'm not, not at all. I'll always love you whatever bad things you've done, and stay with you.' I opened my mouth, Gabriel added: 'and whatever terrible things you do, present or future!' I closed it again.

'Now, would you like a hug?' Gabriel smiles at me properly for the first time this evening.

'Oh yes.'

Gabriel wraps his coat and arms around me, I am enfolded against his heart, I can hear it strongly beating. I'm home. 'Why don't we both sleep on the floor?' I hear myself ask after a while in a muffled voice, then we are both laughing helplessly, if rather hysterically.

****

Romance

The instructor, Luc, complimented the class the following morning. 'If you carry on this well, I think we could try a Red Run tomorrow.' People looked apprehensively at each other. Nell, a young Dutch woman, said reassuringly to Ursula, 'It's a very easy one here, and we'll do the Blue beforehand to work up to it.'

Sure enough, those that wished to, followed Luc down the Red Run during the last forty-five minutes of the morning session. Nell and Ursula skied close together, encouraging each other. Ursula's toes ached with tension by the time she reached the bottom of the slope; she had been scared of falling over. Everyone thoroughly enjoyed it though, and she and Nell were particularly thrilled.

Ali and Jean smiled kindly, as Nell and Ursula rapturously described their morning. In turn, they described the Black Run they'd explored, but encouragingly. 'If you're skiing this well now, you'll be doing the Black Runs before long,' promised Jean.

'Ursula, do you mind if I go off to ski on the other side of the valley with Jean?' asked Ali after they'd had all eaten their croque monsieurs.
'Of course not,' she exclaimed. She enjoyed the time she spent on her own painting or reading.
'I have to go now, too' said Nell, standing up. 'See you tomorrow, Ursula.'
Ursula decided to go down the Red Run again, on her own. She felt a frisson of fear, but if she managed it, what an achievement! She looked forward to telling Nell about it afterwards. Having been silently worried that she would be no good at skiing and might hold the class back, Ursula was secretly thrilled with her progress. She looked at her watch and decided to have another café viennoise in the sun. There was no rush.

It was past four o'clock by the time she reached the top of the Red Run. The sun was sinking lower in the sky, but was still well above the range of mountains. When Ursula steadied herself on her skis and clutched the sticks firmly in gloved hands, the slope looked steeper than it had earlier. Long blue shadows stretched almost across its width. She waited for the few people who had come up on the drag lift with her, to ski down ahead. She needed to take her time.

Half an hour later, Ursula's heart was thudding with fright. She stood frozen with vertigo on the edge of the slope. Her confidence had deserted her after she had fallen, painfully twisting her knee. One ski had flown off, and come to rest about fifty yards further down the mountain. It had taken her twenty minutes to to hobble down to where it rested, and another ten to click the recaltricant ski back onto her boot. Trying not to panic, Ursula estimated she was approximately half-way down the long Red Run. Very few skiers or snow-surfers had passed her, and the sun was sinking behind the mountains. If I get stuck up here in the dark, I'll die of exposure, she thought, breaking out in a cold sweat. She hadn't told
anyone where she'd gone. Even now the authorities were probably closing the lifts, and she needed another drag lift at the end of this run, to be able to get back to the hotel.

She took a shaky breath. It was no good standing here panicking, night was falling, she had to move. Rigid with fear, Ursula slid her skis experimentally forward a little way. Come on, a bit more, she muttered. She began to pep-talk herself through it. A bit more, now you've traversed half-way across the slope, when you get to the other side, turn round before you've thought, because that's the scary bit, when you look down the mountain-' Her words ended in a small scream as a skier narrowly missed her, rocketing past out of nowhere. Ursula shook, wavered and fell, sliding helplessly across icy snow. The person had skidded to a halt further down, and began stepping sideways back up towards her on their skis. As pain tore through her knee, she bit her lip hard and clutched her leg.

'I thought it was you' said Anthony resignedly, looming up beside her.

'You nearly knocked me over,' Ursula said furiously, then spoilt it by bursting into tears.

'I hurt my knee earlier, so I couldn't ski properly, and I'm a beginner' she explained haltingly.

'I couldn't see you, wearing white. You shouldn't be up here when it's almost dark like this' he said gently.

'I know.'

He raised an eyebrow at her tone. 'Now, where does it hurt?' She pointed, watching as his long fingers gently probed her knee.

'Oww!' she gasped.

'I think you've pulled a tendon.' He leant back and unzipped a pocket. 'Have a mint.' She took one, feeling obscurely comforted.

'Now if I help you, do you think you can stand again? We can't stay here.' Ursula nodded. With him she felt safe. Anthony put his arm under hers, and lifted her to her feet. 'Hold on to me' he ordered. Meekly, she held onto his shoulders. He fastened the top button of her ski suit; her skin tingled. She wondered if it was her imagination that he was taking longer than necessary. All her senses were concentrated on his touch, his fingers moved deliberately round to the nape of her neck. Gently he lifted the heavy plait of hair to pull her collar more warmly up round her neck. She felt his fingers lightly brush her throat.

*'Don't you have a hat?' His breath stirred the hair on her
forehead as he concentrated. He smelt clean, and very
slightly of a lemon fragrance.
'No,' she said shakily.
'Well never mind, we'll be down soon. Otherwise I'd undo
your hair.'
Her senses reeled at the thought.
'Why?' she asked neutrally.
'To try and keep your ears warm.'
He impatiently raked a hand through his own dark hair, before
putting his gloves on.*

*'Keep hold of your sticks Ursula, I'm going to undo your ski
bindings.' He moved round behind her, 'Ready?' He kicked
them loose, expertly.
'But why-?' she began again.
'Please trust me, Ursula! Stand in front of me, on my skis.
I'm going to take you down.' She heard the clatter of her skis
as he lifted them on to his shoulder. She stepped forward
reluctantly, looking fixedly at his chest.
'Facing the other way' he said with an undercurrent of
laughter. Blushing, she turned to face outwards. His arm
suddenly closed around her, pulling her back firmly against
him. Ursula gasped as they suddenly accelerated down the
slope. There was no room for fear, her senses were in
turmoil at being held against him. The air was cold against
her face. She could feel his warmth against her back and the
muscles in his thighs were hard against her body, as the skis
beneath them swerved and hissed on the blurred snow. As
they slowed down beside the drag lift she thanked him twice
gratefully, clumsily taking her skis.
'No need to thank me.' He added softly, 'It was most
enjoyable rescuing you.' She looked
up at him quickly to find that he was staring down at her. It
was too dark for her to see his face properly.
'We'll miss the lift' she said breathlessly.
'You have to put your skis on first,' Anthony said slowly. He
held her arm lightly as she stepped onto them, she could feel
the electricity of his touch through her sleeve. She shivered
as he pressed his boot onto the back bindings of her skis.
Misunderstanding her response, he stepped back quickly.
She looked up to see his face had become an impassive*

mask. Feeling dismayed, Ursula slid forward unsteadily, and grabbed at the pole of the drag lift. She was pulled forward along the hill back towards the hotel.

As she limped beside Anthony across the hotel forecourt, he said 'You promise to tell someone next time you have ideas of going off on your own?'
'Yes' said Ursula meekly, feeling an irrational joy at his concern.
'After all' he said briskly 'I won't be around next time to help, we're off to Les Arc 2000 tomorrow.' The arrogance of the man!
'It won't happen again,' she heard herself saying stiffly.

....

Ursula was astonished as they entered the hotel foyer, to see Ali and Celia standing together in the foyer. She could see at a glance that they were not pleased to see her and Anthony together. 'Where have you been?' they demanded almost in unison, as Ursula self-consciously blinked in the bright electric light.
'It's my fault; I tried to do the Red Run on my own, and fell and hurt my knee. T was passing and kindly helped me down.' said Ursula quickly. Celia's face relaxed into a patronising smile, as she looked at Ursula's dishevelled appearance.
'A Red Run?' she said with a little laugh, She linked her arm with Anthony's and he nodded brusquely to Ali, and hardly less so at Ursula as they walked off towards the stairs.

Ursula could not attend the rest of the ski classes to her regret. The hotel doctor strapped up her knee and she spent the next few days outside the mountain cafe, painting. Nell discovered where she was, and came up to see her the first afternoon. Ursula was finishing her second water-colour.
'That's good Ursula! I didn't know you could paint.'
'Well, I don't very often really,' said Ursula, pleased and embarrassed.
'What's happened to you? Are you injured?'
Nell was fascinated when Ursula related a heavily-edited version of what had happened.

'He rescued you? Like a real romance. Is he good-looking?'
she asked teasingly.
'Yes, very' admitted Ursula reluctantly.
'You've got a husband - please pass any surplus handsome
strangers in this direction!' joked Nell. She looked over
Ursula's shoulder again.
'Ursula, you should sell these paintings. In fact I'll buy one if
you have one to spare.'
'No, you can have one,' said Ursula, pleased.
'I'll buy it. It may be worth a lot one day, then I can boast I
paid a pittance for it!' said Nell firmly.
'Anyway, I'd like a memory of this holiday - and Red Runs!'
Nell exploded with laughter, as Ursula flicked water at her.

****

Undine

What the hell has been going on? I feel as though I've been
temporarily deranged. I regressed, I've said the most childish
and embarrassing things to Alex, I mean Alexander. What
was all that about? I'm at an age, almost thirty for goodness'
sake, when I should have shed the dysfunctional elements of
my upbringing, be autonomous. You come from a
dysfunctional family Undine, deal with it. You feel responsible
for it being dysfunctional; I don't think even you could manage
that single-handedly Undine, but if you did, you can't change
the past, only try to keep on an even keel in future. There,
pep-talk to self over. I'm scared.

I took a week off from work following that awful evening, I
think really that Gabriel saved my life. He sat next to me for
moral support when I rang Marco last Thursday from *The Ark*
and said I had domestic problems and asked for Leave to sort
them out. They were very understanding at work.

I feel a bit sorry for Alexander, but he's strong or should be in
his profession. More importantly Gabriel's already had a hard
time due to me, and I feel awful about it, yes 'awful' is the
correct word. I'm going to ring him on the mobile he's given
me right now and tell him how much I love him.

****

Therapy Session

It is most likely that a combination of psychological, biological, environmental and other factors result in the development of the disorder.**

I decided eventually to return to see Alexander, to try and bring about some sort of positive closure. I noticed a leaflet for a psychiatry convention on the table as I passed, heading for the familiar couch.
I wonder what it's like attending an assembly of psychotherapists and psychiatrists? A high percentage of them will have cultivated the tools of the trade, or perhaps it's genetic by now: soft caring voices, automatically nodding heads like those toys for the back shelves of cars and skill at sustaining a disconcerting silence and then asking caringly, 'What do *you* think it means?' No wonder Alexander doesn't have any wrinkles, it's all that practising looking bland so as to be poker-faced when a patient confesses they murdered someone on their way to the session.

What's the term for such a group? Multitude of mental health gurus? Meeting of the mad? Swarm of the self-absorbed? Exhibition of egos? Whatever, everyone present will no doubt be diligently reading body language, making conscious efforts not to script-write or mind-read erroneously – all the while promoting their own reputation, and being careful which words they employ. How exhausting. I bet most of them are people who entered the profession due to trying to sort out their own oddities, or have experienced mental illness somewhere in their family tree... A Nugget of Nutters then.

I was reminded of something: 'Can't I just get hold of the nugget of anxiety inside me that's causing all the rituals and worry and fear, and pluck it out? I asked suddenly, 'Can't we go to the core?'
'No,' Alex looked at me kindly. 'How have you been since I saw you last?'
'Actually, very upset.'
He continued looking for something on his desk.

'Yes?'

'Yes! I was very upset by our last session.' That gained his attention, he came and sat down opposite me, looking surprised.

'I didn't realise, why didn't you ring or email me afterwards?'

'Because I don't like 'phones, as even you should remember, because I don't have easy access to email, but mainly because I seriously considered committing suicide!' Wow. Alexander said: 'My father tried to commit suicide, I saw him, covered in blood, lying on the pavement. I was eleven. He threw himself off a fifth-floor balcony.'

Helplessly I found myself reverting to polite, conditioned-female, sympathetic listener: 'I'm sorry to hear that.'

Doesn't he remember about Grania? Doesn't he remember my real mother died? A pulse of strengthening anger and self-esteem moves suddenly inside me.

....

'Can I just ask you something else?'

Alexander looked reluctant, we'd just decided to concentrate on exposure for the rest of the session.

'People with OCD, are they only hard on themselves about things they're worried whether they've done, or also about things they actually have done that are bad?'

'Both.'

There's a moment's silence. I could tell this charlatan what I did to William, my younger brother, but I no longer feel any need to do so. I can live with this, coping from day to day on my own. I emerged from this epiphany to see Alexander looking furtive.

'You haven't told me what you did have you?' He had the grace to betray a moment's panic. Unforgivable to treat people's traumas that cavalierly. An inept performer, he juggles clumsily with destructive emotions and words. It's like giving a child a box of matches in a firework factory.

'No, Alexander, I haven't.' I regarded him with distaste.

'You could try working out why you did it Undine. I'm going to self-disclose here-'

'You don't have to,' I interrupted. Self-disclose, jargon. Why doesn't he just say like any normal person: 'I'm going to tell you something personal'?

'I think it's appropriate. I did something I'm not proud of when I was a child, to my much younger sister when I was supposed to be looking after her. I stabbed her with a pencil, it hurt her hand badly, thank goodness nothing worse happened. I feel remorse every time I see the scar. I adore my baby sister, we see each other a lot. I can't change what happened. I don't think it has affected her pathologically, but who knows?' He looked sad. 'One can try to understand why one did something like that – I was very unhappy at the time.'

My mind flinched, my act was partly sexually motivated, and also bullying. I was probably unhappy, maybe jealous. I don't remember contentment or feelings of emotional safety occurring much in my childhood. I also worry that I did more to William sexually than I definitely recall. 'Baby sister' as said by Alex makes me feel bad, also unnatural. I never loved my brother in the uncomplicated way that other people seem to love their siblings. Alex feels remorse, but I hit other children viciously, even up to my early teenaged years, some of them much younger than me, when I too was supposed to be looking after them. Looking back on behaviour which would disturb me greatly if I saw a child or teenager manifesting it now, I surmise that it was partly that I lashed out. It was a release from mental torment; also to some extent, bravado - a mixture of the themes I absorbed from old-fashioned books, and the comics I read. It could also have been partly attributed to Grania's behaviour as sometimes she hit us, or partly a form of bullying, although usually unpremeditated. To be physically strong was something to aspire to. Other parents sometimes angrily pointed out the bruising and cuts I'd inflicted on their children, but I never felt anything emotionally. In my teens I worried about whether I'd caused people to die, but or have lasting injuries, but often didn't realise the pain involved in just hurting someone. I thought other people weaklings if they didn't cope. Strangers were often gentle with me, until they experienced my behavioural problems. Often termed ' a nice girl'. I feel, and have felt, guilt, fear and remorse by the ton but it doesn't help anybody.

'I think things may be, very slowly, beginning to move on,' I said to Alexander.
'It comes up a lot in family therapy, what siblings do to each other…' Alexander muttered.

....

I'm not there yet - being compassionate towards myself - although I'm much better than I was.'
'But you will be.'
'You changed my whole picture of myself incidentally, when you said that I was good at dealing with things. I thought, this is something clever you say to people to make them feel better about themselves, *ergo* they cope better.'
'I wouldn't say it if I didn't mean it. You've had a lot to cope with Undine. If you weren't skillful at dealing with things, I would say instead that you're not very good at coping with things yet, but you will be.'
He added, casually: 'You can do anything you like, Undine,' glancing at his wristwatch. For the first time I realised this and not as a threat to myself. Two epiphanies in half an hour! Alexander has given me a rare parting gift that I can reverently look at, turning it shining and safe in my mind.

I smiled at him. I became aware that my fingers were white under the nails because I was holding the folder so hard, containing overspill from my brain. My anxiety began blossoming like some dreadful flower about leaving a trail of words on the cardboard. Stop it, that's an OCD thought. I handed the folder to him, taking care not to look at it and start checking. I rose to leave.

****

Undine

I'm sitting cross-legged on the sitting-room carpet at Einstein Road, but actually on a voyage of discovery. The room's lovely now, with shaded lamps and pictures up on the walls. The fire's crackling cheerfully and I'm surrounded by books. I can touch library books normally now for quite long periods and I only check them once before I return them.

The 'experts' – I'm the real expert of course, being the one with OCD - begin by extolling the virtues of taking serotonin reuptake inhibiting drugs for the condition: 'Although OCD has been recognized for centuries, effective treatment for this condition has been available only for the past four decades. The treatments of choice for OCD are behaviour therapy, consisting of exposure and response prevention, and selective serotonin reuptake-inhibiting medication.'[**]

Apparently Clomipramine is the most widely researched medication, but some mental health professionals state that not enough research has been done, and that drugs aren't great : 'average symptom reduction is only moderate[*] and also don't effect a cure: '... Cure of OCD is not commonplace. The primary goal of treatment in the majority of cases is to have the individual control the disorder rather than the obsessional disorder control the individual.'[***] This theory supports Alexander's belief that there isn't a cure for OCD, just help for people to diminish the symptoms so that they're in charge and the illness doesn't run their lives. Mind you, I heard someone else saying they thought OCD was curable.

In the end I reckon it's best not to get too caught up in all the contradictory theories, I'll just plod onward, tortoise and hare stuff. I've travelled a long way already. Alexander said that I had chronic long-term anxiety too, which fits. What the hell did I do in a past life to be burdened with this?

Having said that, these books are interesting: I've found a paragraph about brain operations, except they term it 'psychosurgical techniques'. Aspiring medical students (paradox or tautology?) could research at least two of these areas, and I've only read the first twenty pages. Apparently the notion that the addition of behavioural therapy to pharmacological treatment may well prevent the relapse associated with cessation of medication, has not been specifically addressed in any study to date. Also, gradually tapering medication as a method of reducing the high relapse rate in OCD sufferers has not been tested in any controlled fashion. How ridiculous, if true, because loads of articles estimate that as many as 1 in 45 people suffer from Obsessive Compulsive Disorder.

I've just read, and wish I hadn't, that in only a third of cases is ECT applied according to medical guidelines considered to be good practice. How awful! Part of the problem is the NHS and other services doing things on the cheap. Perhaps it'll come to buying a kit from a Chemist and doing it ourselves at Einstein Road? I can't wait to hold two electrical wires, with Chloris standing by to break the current with a wooden stick.

That's enough for now, or I won't want to eat the meal I'm about to prepare for supper this evening. We're having a Girlie Evening in and are each bringing a guest, mine's Helena.

****

Torquil

I had a horrible dream that Gabriel sailed away on *The Ark* with Undine; I jumped awake with my heart thumping uncomfortably hard, clad in two jumpers and borrowed track suit bottoms under a sleeping bag on a nylon settee smelling of dogs. Christopher's taste is dreadful. For some reason I don't mind though, I've been staying here for almost a week now. For someone so wealthy, Chris is typically mean, the slut, and won't pay the Cleaner to come in more than once a week. Scared myself to death watching a horror film with him last night, which might account for the nightmare. I decided to leave Chris's place early this morning to check that *The Ark* was still moored to the Pier. I'm trying not to ring Chris, but I've spent half the day riveted to the boat railings looking for his car, because he said he might drop round. First time I've felt like this in a long time, since I met Gabriel in fact. Austin was hilarious in the experimental dance studio before the film on Tuesday, I took Chris round to meet them. I don't know why Brian hasn't told Austin he's too fat for Lycra.

I managed to tear myself away from *The Ark* long enough to go swimming today at the YMCA in town. I wanted to see some friends, but also to have a blissfully hot shower as the water pipe leading from land to the boat has frozen solid. I told Gabriel he should have lagged it better. On the way there, an amusing lift attendant at Russell Square aggrievedly asked this woman to move back so that he could close the doors. We were all jammed in as usual.

'If it had been a real fur coat you was wearing you'd have stood back quicker!'

'It's fake, I've got the hat to match at home, on top of the wardrobe.'

For some reason that made everyone laugh, all trapped in this box. At least now at *The Ark*, we have the multi-fuel stove in the sitting room. It gives out so much heat that we have to throw all the doors and windows open. There's a smell of scorching wood from the underside of the windowsill, three foot from the stove, but the cats are in heaven. Teresa is doing an oil pastel of me naked on Wednesday, as part of her assessed art project. I'll get her to come to the boat, her flat is icy and I want to look my best.

****

Undine

I'm still viewing Alexander in clear, dispassionate, 'daylight'. Of course it was overwhelming that someone has made it their work and seems to have some comprehension of my OCD, but it's also an illusion. They don't really, not an insider's view. He was just a tool, ultimately a boring one at that, to try and shift the tedious rituals, the banal frustrating compulsion that's kept me staring at things, or at surprised strangers. Not really seeing them, the taps that is, that's the sad thing: otherwise there would be all these obsessive-compulsive new post-Naturalist artists. Also photographers, who would aim to show the atoms shifting within the chrome. They could open a Starck II designer paradise in Chelsea. Society would fete the 'mad' creator, this time while they were still alive for a change.

****

Alexander

Lucy was strange when I returned home this evening; it had been a long day. I'd seen thirteen different patients, fitting my lunch into twenty minutes, very lucrative. Exhausting though, so I wasn't really up to par. Initially I thought Lucy was cross because I was only just in time to say good-night to Louisa, my little treasure, and tuck her in. But when I went downstairs, to open a bottle of red wine for us to drink with dinner, Lucy turned from the table and silently held out a folded sheet of white paper. It felt like a Summons.

'What's this?' I set down the bottle and corkscrew on the sideboard and foolishly took it.

'I imagine it's a *billet doux* from Wendy, I don't know why you kept it in your jeans pocket, but I don't much care.'

I stared at her, 'But Wendy's no longer my Supervisor,' was all I could think of to say. Lucy sighed. I noticed that she was unusually pale, there were shadows under her eyes and her mouth was set in a thin disillusioned line. She's in danger of losing her looks.

'You forget that you only work at the end of the street, Alexander. Benedict heard part of your recent conversation with Wendy as he passed. A pity you had to hold it on the doorstep.'

'Oh, but she's off her rocker.' I laughed. 'I think the menopause's arrived early, she's begun entertaining all sorts of strange ideas. That's why I asked to be transferred to a different Supervisor.'

'Wendy is, was, pregnant.'

'Is she?'

Was?

'Yes, I took the liberty of 'phoning her at work and we met this morning. It was very enlightening.'

'What makes her, or you, think it was mine?'

'Alexander-' Lucy struggled with words for a moment then articulated painfully: 'You've betrayed me again, we've only been together for four years for God's sake! And you did it here, where we live!'

For a horrible second I thought Lucy knew about the fun and games in the dining-room - surely Wendy hadn't told her that - but then I realised she was just upset because Benedict had cottoned on. With that she left the room and I heard her heavily climbing the stairs. She hadn't cooked any supper. I 'phoned for an Indian takeaway and tried to think what to do. Why do difficulties always arise when one's really tired? I suddenly remembered the sheet of paper and unfolded it, perplexed. It was quite a saucy love poem ostensibly from Wendy to Peter Pan, Lucy's pet name for me, although not for a while now. Suddenly understanding dawned. Undine. Undine's bloody writing! I'd chucked away the other thing she'd written – I couldn't be bothered to read it - but must have forgotten to look in the other pockets when throwing my jeans at the laundry bin. Not like me. So I was right about Undine; she entertained naughty notions - little bitch. How the hell was I going to sort out this mess? I'd managed it before, but more was called for this time. Better take Lucy on a 5-star holiday, she's hinted about the Bahamas enough times. Expensive though. Come to think of it, her pal Toby still has a place there ... Around midnight I fell asleep on the sofa, with the television on. When I woke stiff-necked and groggy at eight the next morning, Lucy had left me, taking the Lotus and Louisa to her all-powerful Mummy and Daddy.

Well at least I know my job pretty well now, thanks to Wendy. I'll need to set up somewhere else though. The consulting room and basement were rented cheap through Harry, but he was Lucy's friend. The Old Girls' Network we called it.

****

Gabriel

I love the way Undine makes different humming noises when she's cleaning her teeth. She's stayed with me several times since *that* night, I think Torquil is at Chris's boat. The brushing, loosely translated, can be heard as: 'up down, once across, once up right, down one right, once up left, down twice right [expectorate into basin] 'down twice left upper, across twice.' If I make her giggle she starts all over again, so now if I hear her I just listen fondly from the hall.

From what Florence was saying, it sounds as though my Temp assignment will definitely finish the end of the second week of January as Lasain is actually doing some work instead of sloping off early, and interviewing victims for my post. Although I'll be relieved to stop doing unconducive work, I'll really miss Florence and Maisie, most people in the hospital unit in fact. I'll buckle down this week to lining up auditions to attend, in case I slump into unemployment. I end up getting more done when I'm working, fitting in social and domestic activities around the job, than when an empty day yawns.

****

Therapy Session

Alexander's persuaded me, I'm not sure how which is disconcerting, to attend a couple of final sessions of what I call aversion therapy and he terms 'exposure'. Anyway, it means none of my distracting anecdotes about other areas of my life and mental landscape, we have to buckle down to it. This sounds very straightforward until I arrive on his doorstep and have a panic attack. I reel dizzily along the hall, and into the sitting-room. When I can speak properly, I blurt resentfully: 'Can you teach me to make myself relax? It shouldn't be that I need you to make me feel better when this happens.'

I suddenly realise that he looks awful. Alexander, of all people, looks rough! He looks as though he's slept in his clothes. His eyes are red-rimmed, he reeks of smoke and there's a grey tinge to his tanned face. When the magic stopped this is what he turned into: the picture of Dorian Gray. 'Are you all right?' I ask.
'Yes.' He's curt. 'Shall we do some breathing?'
'Breathing doesn't really work for me. And I couldn't manage deep breathing at all right now.'
'I get people who are about to perform to thousands of people to use this breathing to calm themselves down, and it works!'
Huh.
I count six self-consciously and slowly aloud, as instructed, for him to breathe in, then 12 for him to breathe out.
He does it for me, then I do it myself for a while he scribbles.
I do feel more relaxed, partly because of the silence, apart from the faint sibilance of my breath. Iris stopped breathing when no-one was there. By the time she died, her personality

had been smashed by the drugs used to counteract the worst effects of the Cancer which ate her alive. I feel my expression waver and then there are tears all over my hands and I can hear that Alex has stopped writing.
'Sorry,' I say after a while. He doesn't ask me what I'm upset about.

We start with taps, as we've done some exposure therapy with them before. I know you haven't read about it, but I don't relate everything that happens in my life, you have to watch reality TV, read books or live with friends for that. I march in and out of the bathroom, opening the door, turning the light on, turning the taps on full, turning them off, looking at them once to ensure that they're off. If they're not fully off, then the house-owner should call in a plumber, their problem. I turn off the light, being ecologically-minded, and return to my seat without looking back. Actually, being watched for part of this is both daunting and reassuring, I feel self-conscious about my body, even though Alexander is punctilious about not looking below the ears. Odd that, the self-consciousness I mean, as I lost these inhibitions a few years ago when I became much more relaxed about my appearance. I've noticed that I've also started biting my tongue again and worrying about whether I've talked aloud about my anxieties when alone, and I'm standing on the scales, wondering if earrings count – only once every two days – but obviously OCD has reared up for its Last Stand. It can desperately yank out all the old patterns of behaviour it likes, the bastard. It's not going to win this time. I just have to be on my guard.

After the fifth time of turning taps on and off, I'm complaining that I'm bored. (I also think that this has limited usefulness as an exercise, as having someone present is reassuring and I need to learn to do it on my own.)
'I don't care.' Alexander said brusquely. I thought that was brilliant, much better than all that pseudo-caring bullshit. I think that's been one of the things that's been hard to handle: loads of 'caring', thinly covering scientific interest and profiteering. I don't know what NHS work Alexander's done in the past, if any, but he doesn't accept NHS referrals now. Rather hypocritical of me when I've been subscribing to private medicine, but I'll go through the NHS now that I can

cope better, even if I have to wait months for an appointment. I'm not sure how well I'll manage being 'clinicalised' or whatever the word is, though. I think I'll check it all out with Chloris or BACUP first.

'I know you don't care,' I said happily to Alexander. And that was it, spell broken. He looks smaller than I remember. He's only human, whereas Gabriel now ... Gabriel is an Angel.

Which is what enabled me later in the session, via touching table surfaces and the brocade of the hall chair, to be kneeling indifferently only centimetres from Alexander, on the hall floor. I was feeling the underneath of the large wooden table in the hall busily with my fingers, as was he. As you know from reading this far, one of my manifestations of OCD has been the dread of touching inanimate objects in places that I won't be able to check easily afterwards. Yes, I know it's not logical, but the fact that I realise this means I'm not mad. Get it?

It is weird, paying a stranger to indulge in the same strange behaviour as me, to try and help me overcome it. I won't let myself be upset by this though. Alexander kept asking me what my anxiety levels were. I was so overwhelmed by the whole experience that I was finding it difficult to apply something that seemed so irrelevant.
If I could get my anxiety level down to 5 out of 10, he repeated patiently, then I'd be let off touching the wood any longer. You don't know how tempting it was to say 'Five!' and run out of the house, down the street, catch a 'plane and never, ever see Alexander again. Try and understand – that's why you've read this far. I'll bet you're scared of snakes, right? Imagine if someone dropped one down your back. I personally am not scared of snakes, but I'm not about to crow.

I hope my brain gets used for something useful and career-advancing soon. What a waste of time, fear, grey cells and effort, these rituals are! I'm very glad that the hidden agonising and rumination has improved though, it's so much harder to manage. Don't get me wrong, it's still present, but much less so. Forget 'Je ne regret rien', I do the new version:

'Je regret tous'. If I was given any wish, it would be to become happy in my own skin.

I asked him if we'd be feeling the underneath of armchairs during the next session. I was scared. Alexander said 'Yes,' then seemed to come to a decision. He said that the lease was up on this room as the owner was suddenly selling up and that he was looking for new premises to work from. He said that it shouldn't mean too much of a delay and could he notify me as soon as he had his new address? I was shocked.
'Um yes, fine. How long do you think it'll be?' But even as I asked, on Automatic-Anxiety, I calmed myself. I had privately dispensed with Alexander's services, if the need arose I could consult someone else. But how many psychotherapists *et al* are more screwed up than their patients? I looked at Alexander with pity, and he hated it. I glimpsed venom for a second before the indifferent mask slid back into place.

****

Gabriel

Apparently the boat needs re-insuring. I wouldn't mind but Kirsty got wind of it somehow and says if it's not insured then the boat has to be moved from the mooring. It'd be really hard to find a new mooring in London; I've heard there are only 250 altogether and waiting lists. The trouble is, the last time I rang round, no-one wanted to ensure the poor old Ark. I bet Noah didn't have these problems. I might ask Finn if there's anything going up at Camden Lock, I'd be near Undine then too.

For several days, 'planes have been re-routed away from their normal flight paths over the pontoon, due to a strong easterly wind. The opposite happened following the American war-mongering in Iraq: planes weren't flown over central London, but circled above the pontoon instead. This noise, added to the usual Police and traffic-reporting helicopters - which when flown too low made you feel as though you're playing the lead in *Apocalypse Now* while having a cup of tea in the sitting-room – meant that the boat vibrated constantly for weeks. Torquil and Chris have almost convinced me that if planes had crashed in Chiswick, just as many people would have died as in the centre of town. The boys look quite sweet together; Torquil joking about moving to Chelsea hasn't extended to him seriously considering moving the cats, but I don't mind. I like having them around, so does Undine. She has banned them from the bedroom though and as they hardly ever scratch at the door now, she must have more cat-cred than me. She's asked Chris if I can give a presentation of my inventions, particularly the one of customized KittyKlean trendy cat flaps. If they could be manufactured and sold, it would be great.

****

Romance

In the evenings, Ursula was fussed over during the apres-ski gatherings now taking place in the Bar. While everyone around her enthusiastically drank and related their progress on the ski slopes, she listened and resisted offers of beer, and other more flirtatious offers. Ursula blossomed. She felt as though she was now enjoying a youthful time she hadn't been able to before. She avoided alcohol: both her parents had drunk rather too much at different times and she liked to be in command of herself. Perhaps she had exercised too much control and caution, Ursula sometimes thought. Never mind, her life was opening up enough now.

Towards the end of the holiday, Ursula began to consider putting together her sketches and paintings into a portfolio. Several people had now commented favourably on her work. She remembered that there were a lot of canvases tucked away in a large cupboard - some she hadn't looked at for several years. Maybe she could even exhibit them somewhere? It would be wonderful to earn money from something she enjoyed doing so much. Sorry as she would be to leave the Alps, she looked forward to returning to London.

****

Undine

Undine listened; all she could hear was a bird singing and
intermittent sawing of wood, as Dion made a bench outside in
the cleared back garden. Sunlight lay on the faded tiles on
the passage floor. The door to the spare room was ajar, she
glanced at the clean vacant room. Rosalie had departed two
days before. They'd held a leaving party for her, Undine had
taken pleasure in helping Matilda and Chloris to organise it,
as well enjoying the actual event itself. She'd designed the
invitations, a cartoon of them all at the house, and
photocopied them - as well as preparing food for the buffet
without worrying whether she was contaminating it with germs
or broken glass. She'd been having a sad month, but still, it
made her realise that she was conquering the OCD. The
house had been alive with friends' laughter, food, flirtation and
music.

Now Undine flexed her hands, sighed, then suddenly
crouched down to open the last notebook in the cardboard
box.

****

Torquil

I'm staring at an illicit fag-end rolling between the slats on the
floor, while the Tube train snorts its way up the pale blue line
from Brixton. Our nostrils were powdery from the white lines
at the party (does that excuse me?) A momentary aberration,
but I love you Gabriel, I do! I thought you were gay, I still
think you are, you just can't deal with it. What about all those
times we used to meet in the pulsating, sweating air in the
basement of The Arches? The first time we saw each other, I
thought what a smooth white forehead you had and gorgeous
voice. We didn't speak, we were jealous of each other. We
used to meet each other by chance exactly an hour late on
Hungerford Bridge – everyone else used to be kept waiting
but some sort of telepathy operated with you. What about all
those times you took my men – not that, but they all made
eyes at you over my shoulder while we chatted. You used to

depend on me: 'Torquil! It's me, chuck down the keys,' you shouted down in the street, you sounded desperate, and you were. Some conniving trollop had told you you'd got her up the duff. It was me who found out she was lying, for you.

That bitter winter in Cambridge when I vacated hot comfy room at Halls of Residence in London to come and spend Christmas with you. The bog froze over and snow drifted in through the broken sash window onto the bathroom floor. Everyone huddled round the gas fire in the vast Victorian sitting-room in our coats and boots and smoked. I gave you a tin I liked, and you didn't, for Christmas. I got into my sleeping bag on the floor of your tiny bedroom and stared up at the hideous red paper lampshade and then in the middle of the night, frozen, crawled into bed with you and took all the duvet. When I woke up, you were awake, lying there with no covers in your old flannel shirt, staring uncomplainingly at the ceiling. Apparently I'd tried to cuddle you in my sleep. You'd laid awake for a while wondering what else was going to happen, then relaxed and gone back to sleep. So trusting.

I'm sitting next to you but I daren't look at your white face reflected in the black window. The wires on the underground tunnel wall are orange, purple and yellow, lit by blue flashes thrown up from the rails. I don't know what to say. Oh well, it's all experience. I've got such a headache, but I'm grateful for the noise in here as we career headlong beneath the city, it means I don't have to listen to your deafening silence.

It seemed like such a fun idea last night, I really thought you were up for it. How did I forget that you'd told me you were in love with Undine? I suppose I couldn't believe it, not with her. I never saw anything in her at all, but then I wouldn't. You said you were sorry, you didn't want to - thank God you got away Gabriel. You were pale and strange, I thought you were going to be sick. You do understand that I only wanted you Gabriel, don't you? I'm so sorry.

****

Undine

Thank you, Good Powers that be. I'm breathlessly on my way to the boat now as a surprise. Gabriel will be really pleased as I thought I'd have to work all day, but I managed to get loads of work finished this morning, so Marco gave me the afternoon off. (We're going in on Saturdays at the moment because of the huge Clerkenwell project.) I've texted Gabriel a message on his mobile. The bag of fruit I've just bought is bumping gently against my left thigh as I hurry along. I'm carrying apples so that Gabriel can teach me how to make *Tart Tatin*: I have some really creative ideas for the *entrée* …

It's not long now until Christmas. I've been thinking about what to buy for Gabriel, we're going to spend Christmas Eve together. He invited me to visit his family with him, but I'm not quite ready for that yet, especially at Christmas which I used to find difficult with all its loving family connotations. I've promised to go with him to meet them in the Spring.

****

Gabriel

Oh hell, my mobile was stolen along with everything else that happened at that damned party.

I tersely borrow Torquil's phone and ring Linda to find out if she found anyone to feed the cat this week-end, that way I can avoid Torquil while he moves out. I don't bear him ill-will, but I don't want him around. He's got the message: I've never seen him so subdued. I'll call Undine when I get to Linda's.

****

Gabriel

The bath is filling fast; the problem is that I've locked myself out, venturing briefly into the back garden to coax Doris the cat to savour the morning air. Linda was great when I arrived last night. She could tell something awful had happened, but just looked at me sympathetically as she gave me a spare set of keys. She gets up at the crack of dawn to go to work.

Things have gone with a bang so far this morning; the back door of the house extension slammed and the old-fashioned iron bolt on the bottom dropped neatly into the catch in the concrete floor. Doris rocketed across the blackened, frosty garden, so mission accomplished in that quarter. Unfortunately I wasn't wearing warm space gear, only yesterday's shirt which only just covered extremities and Linda's bedroom slippers in the form of fluffy dogs – unsuitable attire for nervously straddling a rusty fence en route to the octagenarian neighbour's back door. After a lot of loud knocking, an approaching figure could be seen dimly rippling through the frosted glass. 'Yes?' Mrs Moor mumbled, having left her teeth upstairs in the rush and clutching her candlewick dressing gown round her.

She stared at my attire and suddenly gums were bared in helpless wheezing laughter, it was quite alarming. Her matching pink hair hair rollers wobbled with joy. To my mind, it was a moot point which of us appeared the more ridiculous.
'I'm sorry to bother you Mrs Moor. I've locked myself out, have you any keys for next door?'
'No, Duck,' she spluttered.
'Well the bath's filling up in there, so I guess I'd better break the glass in the back door?'
'Good luck dear, you don't want to be out for long in this weather.'
She shut the door briskly, and stumped callously back to her warm and cosy bed. Back over the fence, with pubic hairs standing on end with fright and cold. Doris was sitting purring on the concrete path bisecting the long grassy garden. Panicking I stared around, looking for something with which to effect entry into the house before water poured out of a window into the garden. The only useful thing I could see was an old broom propped against the wall. Nerving myself, I bashed the pane of glass hard. The broom handle bounced off, sending a shock up my arm. Doris stopped washing a hind leg to stare up at me irritably.
'Armoured glass!' I whispered incredulously, Linda was normally so lax about security.

'End justifies the means, Doris.' I charged at the door as though jousting for my life. There was a deafening explosion, an airborne cat and I was covered in fragments of broken glass. I peered through the hole and reached downward gingerly. I couldn't reach the bolt without disembowelling myself on the edge of the window. I could almost hear the bath water building up on top of the first floor ceiling. Oh the relief, there was a bucket by the hedge! It took a long minute to remove the metal curved handle. I reached downward through the broken window and hooked up the bolt with it. I took the stairs two at a time, I couldn't hear water running. This was because the water had reached the bottom of the taps. Just in time.

****

Undine

I'm knocking on the front door of *The Ark*; the sky is cloudy and it's beginning to snow again. The tide is going out and I can see the lamp shining through the blinds of the sitting-room. I'm so excited at the thought of seeing Gabriel that I'm standing on tip-toe on the doormat.

The door is eventually opened, releasing a welcome wave of heat, by Torquil. I'm quite shocked to see that he's only wearing a towel, then see a woman unsmilingly holding a drawing board. He slouches, holding onto the half-open door slightly above me, as I stand on the deck.
'Hi Torquil, is Gabriel back?'
'No.'
'Oh,' I feel a bit odd, he's still standing in the doorway and not moving aside to let me into the warm room. I can see the cats stretching and climbing off the sofa to come and greet me.
'Um, do you mind if I come in and wait in his room for him?' I smile up at him. He smiles back, but unpleasantly.
'To be honest, I'm a bit surprised you're here Undine.'
'Why?' I begin to feel frightened, my feet are freezing.
'Hasn't Gabriel 'phoned you?'
'No, what about?'

'About the party we went to together last night. You know, it doesn't seem right that he's left it to me to tell you.'
'No. I'll ask him myself.'
'Good luck. Let's just say it was a gay party and he had a *very* good time. He's with his new friend right now.'
'I don't believe you.'
Torquil shrugged and sighed. I bent down to hide my burning face and stroked Camberwell who was leaning against my legs, mewing. As I stepped down on to the crate, snow swirled around me and I slipped, landing painfully on the icy pontoon on my knees. I heard the woman say something and Torquil snigger as he shut the front door.

****

Gabriel

When I wake in the early hours, to keep my thoughts diverted I listen to the World Service. I've noticed that whenever they pronounce the full name of a worthy public institution on the radio, it's invariably because the initials spell something embarrassing: I think that's why they added 'severe' and made it 'SARS'. Radio is entertaining, apart from broadcasting increasingly graphic descriptions of gore, particularly in the small hours. Not to mention broadcasters' erroneous usage of singular and plural – but I must stop this carping or I'll become a bore. A male broadcaster on Radio 3, probably embittered by never having made it into the school choir, referred disparagingly the other day to: 'A feisty if not over-reflective performance', by a female opera singer - to me she sounded heavenly. At four o'clock this morning, the announcer said soothingly: 'If you think you have a problem with sex addiction, call the radio helpline' [and someone will come and visit you in your own home in the interests of research]. It was like the Neighbourhood Watch Newsletter: 'Wishing you a very merry Christmas and a peaceful New Year from all the officers of the Police Division' [but not too peaceful or we'll be out of a job, Sir].

It's 4.30am now and I've given up the struggle to sleep. I'll draw up presentation plans for the trendy cat flaps. Insomnia would strike now: I've got the audition as a vet for a new TV series at nine-thirty this morning. I called Undine last night but her mobile seems to be switched off. I tried her at Einstein Road and Matilda, I think it was, said she hadn't seen her but would leave a message.

On the radio, Cornelia Parker said she'd like a solar-powered vibrator on her desert island. It's lucky it's specifed as a 'desert' island, we're sitting on an island here (if you discount the Channel Tunnel) and it's a bleak pastel-hued December day. I'm going up to see my parents for Christmas Day and Boxing Day, the whole clan are gathering there. I must buy present for my nephews and nieces. I wish Undine was coming, I'll miss her. I'll take her shopping on Christmas Eve so that she can choose whatever she likes as her present, but I'll also make her a gift.

****

Undine

I have a very clear recollection of many childhood things; like Peter Pan it was age I did not wish to leave. I wish I hadn't now, I'm not very good at being an adult. I wanted to play hide-and-seek, climb trees and explore the countryside for ever. The beautiful twilight over the dusky fields, the Thames flowing slowly between water meadows, the Downs curving gently in the distance.

Further along the track outside our gate, was the Slaughter House, which was closed down when I was a bit older. Children from the village used to go and play in its shadowy buildings that smelt of something odd: strange and dank. We climbed up onto the high, broken, tiled roofs, or down into the open, deep, water-filled manhole drains. It was always cold inside, even on the hottest Summer day. The huge meat-hooks hung, still and rusting, illuminated by rays of sunlight poking through the holes in the roof.
'We make our common supplication unto thee', squealed the ghosts of pigs as they were herded terrified and running beneath the sharp shining hooks.

My earliest memory was of my Mum's crystal stopper from a scent bottle, she made rainbows on the wall with it when the sun shone. My father saying: 'Your memory!' But I thought he liked me remembering things about my mother, and his mother. He still always prefaces sentences with: I don't expect you remember,' but I always do, sometimes better than him. Perhaps I feel I can control the past, even though memories have almost destroyed me. This handle on the past but not on the present is unhealthy and unnecessary; I need to live in the present. Mum used to laugh though.

I'm realising that sentimentality and nostalgia are for the young. Mature people live pragmatically in the present, divesting themselves of superfluous status symbols, memories and clutter.

....

My new room in the squat in Camden Road is low and large, with old wooden painted 'stable' doors with big iron bolts leading to the overgrown garden. I would have loved it before. One of the worse things was the way in which Torquil looked so gleefully malicious when he told me about that party, and what Gabriel did there. I brushed the floor and walls of my new abode in a storm of dust and oily soot, to try and forget what he said, then washed all the paintwork down with hot soapy water and some old tea-towels that I found in a cupboard. I can't stop crying. Torquil was so matter-of-fact, Gabriel must have been too scared to tell me himself, so asked him to. I rang Gabriel's mobile immediately, although why would Torquil lie? But a stranger answered and swore at me. At least, I hope it was a stranger. Of course it was, Gabriel doesn't swear.

If I leave the oven on, it takes the dank chill off the room. Some of my books, clothes and cosmetics are still at *The Ark*. I bet Torquil is there washing his bleached hair with my camomile shampoo, using a cup over the sink, scrawny torso suspended. I can't face going back. I'll return to Einstein Road next week; thank goodness work is so busy at the moment, it leaves me less time to think. I must have improved: at one time I couldn't work if I was in a state, because I prioritised the miseries. I'm going to save for a trip to the countryside, I need to see the night sky and stars. I saw the moon in my mirror the other evening, so it was confusingly in the wrong place.

****

Gabriel

I'm glad I've inherited the cats: the loneliness would be intolerable otherwise. I keep 'phoning and texting Undine, but she hasn't rung back. If she can't manage the 'phone, I wish she'd write to me. I went to Einstein Road immediately I learned that Torquil had lied to her about the party, but she'd moved out. Matilda and Chloris obviously know where she's gone, but wouldn't say. I could see that they wanted to, but they'd obviously been sworn to secrecy, I wish I had friends that loyal. I've even been to Hammersmith Mall and seen Villainous Vic, but he hasn't heard from Undine. I'll go mad soon if I don't find her, or just know that she's all right. It was Finn who told me about her OCD, he obviously thought I knew.

I braved the West End yesterday for new shoes, almost bought Wellingtons. In obliging pathetic fallacy mode, the sky was weeping big opulent tears onto Oxford Circus. Everything - buildings, streets, vehicles, disgruntled populace - was dirty, soaked, grey and blurred. The latter were being particularly aggressive with their umbrellas. The scraping windscreen wipers on the 94 bus home couldn't keep the streaming windscreen clear, and the interior of the bus smelt of wet wool and iron.

****

Torquil

'I was exhausted afterwards, but I'm going to do it again next Christmas, it's good fun.'
Julian said: 'I couldn't do it, I think you two are saints.' He took a sip of white wine.

I silently concurred, and smiled modestly. I took my own rubber gloves into the homelessness Shelter: red, with holly sprig pattern and fake fur cuffs, they matched my Santa hat.
'Oh no,' that's my unassuming Christopher, looking uncomfortable. 'There but for the grace of God...'
'I see it as woolly-minded, liberal Guardian-reading sentiments run with military precision.' I concluded, rather cleverly I thought.
'You'd think after seeing some of these poor people in such a state from alcohol ... But all the volunteers ended up getting rat-arsed at the local pub after the last shifts, apparently they do at the party too. We'll let you know next week,' offered Chris.
'More Brussels?' asked Nat, passing the tureen.
'Yes please.'
'Deelish meal, thanks Chris and Torquil,' said Nat raising his glass.
'Hear, hear. Happy New Year everyone!' said Julian. He's so handsome. If I wasn't with Christopher... Julian broods better than Colin Firth.
'Oh funny story... Funny story everyone!' I called as we put down our glasses. 'My friend Catherine, she helped me tidy away breakfast on the first day. She was singing carols with other volunteers in the Main Shelter, they were quite good but their voices were getting a bit lost. The place was huge, a massive warehouse this year, and what with the noises off, of shouting, applause and people joining in... Anyway, this man, the dirtiest in the place, bare feet, no teeth, he lurched up to Catherine while she's giving the descant her all, and growled 'Give us a kiss Darling!' and poked his tongue in her ear.'
Shrieks of mirth. 'Gives a whole new dimension to aural sex!'
'Well, as Catherine said: ' I want to make the guests happy over Christmas, but not that happy.' She and I used to text each other competing as to how quickly we could get into the shower after getting home.
'Who won?'
'I did, just. Thirty seconds.'
'Actually, hardly any of the guests are dirty, and you only won because you left your manky clothes all over the floor on the way.' Christopher is improving on the house-cleaning front, a bit.

'What were your favourite jobs? I might do it next year,' That was Nat, acting as peace-maker.

'I liked looking after the stray dogs,' said Chris. Rather him than me, I went out there to see him during my break, and he was walking this quarrelsome little black and white mongrel round the concrete compound in a biting wind, keeping it away from the other dogs and playing with it with a rubber bone. And he had to clean up doggy-doos.

'What about you Torq?'

'The luggage store. There's this really efficient card system to stop people's possessions getting lost. Most of them are in black plastic bags you see. I think in the past sometimes they got thrown out with the rubbish. Then of course all hell breaks loose. Did you do the fag-run, Chris?'

'The what?' asked Julian, eyebrows in his hair.

'Oh you take all these roll-ups that people sit making round a couple of tables in the volunteer section, a good social job that, plus some 'real' cigarettes, out onto the floor and distribute one to everyone who asks. You have to keep them under your jacket, it's like being a spiv: 'Pssst, want a ciggie?' Then the word spreads and if you're not careful you get mobbed. 'Can I have one for my mate, he's in the shower?' You have to be ever so strict and say, 'No, I need to see your mate.'

'I was no good at rolling cigarettes,' said Chris. 'They were either so tight the guests went purple pulling on them, or too loose so that all the tobacco fell out when they held them upright.'

'So that's why I saw some of them wetting their fingers and dabbing at the tables as I followed you round.'

'Some of them asked for 'proper' cigarettes instead, roll-ups were seen as less prestigious.'

'Suzy was nice wasn't she? Did you get her email?'

'Yes, she was good on the main gate, so tactful. That guy she frisked who kept coming back for more!'

'Why do you have to frisk them?' asked Nat, through a mouthful of chicken.

'Because: no weapons, no violence, no drugs, no alcohol,' Chris and I sang in unison.

'Which meant that we later found a neat line of beer cans outside the fence, stretching for yards, hidden in the bushes.'

'With names like 'Stan' scratched on them, with the level of
beer marked!'
There were lots of funny moments, weren't there?' Chris
stood up and began collecting plates.
'I'm not volunteering to work in the Volunteer's
Accommodation year, some of them were real pigs!'
'Now, who's ready for home-made Christmas Pudding?'

****

Gabriel

I'm really pissed off. I'm in Tescos searching for organic,
free-range bacon, all I can see is wall-to-wall special offers for
nudging-sell-by-date brandy butter. It's no good them
assuring me that organic means free-range, I don't believe
them unless they've been forced to print it on the wrapper.
I'm not eating some poor creature that lived and died in Hell.
I know, I need a holiday: impending unemployment is not the
same thing. The hospital job ends the Friday after next. I
was touched when I overheard Florence and Maisie planning
Leaving Drinks for me in the hospital bar. We're going to stay
in touch, they want to visit me on the boat but I've put them off
until March, by which time I'll have done more work on *The
Ark*. When I stepped down from the deck yesterday onto the
upturned beer crates, my foot went through one and frost
thawing on the roof trickled down into my hair.

The real reason I'm hacked off is that, on top of missing
Undine, some bastard nicked my best bike last night. I'd
arranged to meet up with Liam and Matthew at Pickwicks
Wine Bar in an effort to cheer up. I was a bit early so hung
around the High Road and locked my bike to a stand outside
some shops. I ended up buying two books in Waterstones
and five in the discount book shop further along the road, as
well as two DvDs - it's expensive, socialising. A group of
boys were swooping across Chiswick High Road and the
pavement, wearing black clothes on un-lit bicycles, playing
chicken with the traffic. It reminded me that I'd been knocked
down by a car when I'd just put a new halogen lamp on my
bike, so they were chancing it. The motorist swore he didn't
see me - obviously needed a Braille steering wheel.

Liam was in good form, and I began to feel better, to the point of glimpsing emotional normality: the red wine helped. Jonathan arrived, and we adjourned to the Italian restaurant on the corner. I sent my pasta back via a camp Northern waiter, as being too salty. The replacement dish was worthy of Dead Sea status and the cook gave me a malevolent look as I lurched to the Gents. Matthew and Liam still left a tip, middle-class habits die hard. When we went to collect my bike on the way back to the boat for coffee though, it wasn't there. For a couple of minutes I even wondered if I'd remembered correctly where I'd left it. Eventually I gave up searching the High Road and began wending my homeward. Liam and Matthew caught up with me, triumphantly waving my new Remot-Loc in pristine condition. They'd found it looped round a lamp-post near the Tube station. I bet either one of the Black Panthers, or the restaurant Chef, is riding my Cove Hummer. It's only used on special occasions or *in extremis*, and I bought it last year with the final proceeds of the sit-com. I hope the thief becomes Chicken Curry, but that my Hummer is spared.

The wooden pontoon despite being ridged is very slippery – have visions of myself stepping out of the front door and skidding straight into the Thames. The sunrise was bloody and beautiful this morning, Undine would like it. I'll take a photo and make a card and send it to her by old-fashioned post. A new start.

****

Torquil

'I love you.'
'I know.'
'Oh why do you have to be so calm? When I've said that to other people they – oops!'
'And how long did they last?'
'Point taken. How would you like your eggs done this morning Christopher Robin? Sunny side up?'
'Yes please. Have you rung Gabriel yet to apologise?'
I slammed the 'fridge door.

'Have you Torquil?'

'No.'

Silence.

'Oh all right! I'll do it today, it's just… difficult and I'm scared to talk to Gabriel. What if he won't speak to me? I feel so bad already, being so happy with you, when I've split them up.'

'I know, but I'm here for you, although it's more than you deserve.'

I carried breakfast up into into the wheel-house. I'd garnished the plates beautifully. I put them down carefully on the table as inspiration struck.

'Chris, I know, I know what to do!'

'Good.' He picked up a fork.

'I could, we could, search for Undine and tell her I lied. I mean, find her properly.'

'We?'

'You will help, won't you?'

'Oh all right. Now let's have breakfast, we'll talk about it later. Pass me *The Independent* please, without sticking your nose in it.'

'Here you are, do you like the flowers I bought?'

'Yes.'

****

Gabriel

I'm on my way to the Vet Audition. Traversing across London Bridge after alighting at a dilapidated station. Staring down through a broken window onto the track and platform and roof. A man was adjusting his clothing by an old wooden fence, thinking himself unobserved. There's a smell of iron and wood as I thump down steps. Through windows on the left, I catch an incongruous glimpse of scruffy Nature. On this sunny cold morning, I look back under the lofty, curved, glass and iron roof, and see the sunlight glinting and hazy across thousands of heads. Receptacles of thoughts, exhaustion, zest for life, ambition, excitement, awe, depression or pride – the warm light bestowing an indifferent Benediction. Despite missing Undine, and to some extent, bloody Torquil, my heart lifts at the contagious energy of London. Buses roar around the corners under a railway bridge to the left. Trains shunt across as we swing onto the bridge, the shuffle and tramp of feet – an array of individuals. On across the bridge marching with thousands of others, past the silvered lion standing on his hind legs bearing an heraldic shield. Past too the astounding height, blasphemously higher than a church tower, of the glass and marbled arch of corporate cathedral, No. 1 London Bridge. Ornamental plants on external ledges, a lone cleaner swaying in his giddy box, cleaning the shell of the modern monolith. The wide Thames is gelatinous and green-grey, rocking the toy HMS Belfast down near Tower Bridge.

The customary beggar, a pale young man with a blanket around him intoning politely: 'Have a good day, change please' like a stuck CD, his back against the icy stone balustrade. Trains like primary-coloured caterpillars. An aeroplane overhead. Sky an ethereal blue above the 'Gherkin' – architecture by Foster, backdrop by God. Red double-decker buses swing out round corners, car engines roar, pneumatic drills ring, a Police launch passes beneath us on the river. A necklace of lights follows the curve of the river bank. On the left St. Paul's Cathedral shines in the mist, dwarfed by buildings like the two towers on the opposite side of our bridge. They evoke the massive Fascististic copies of the Campanile at the entrance to Barcelona's Olympic Stadium. London is alive and vibrant, oh yes!

The curve of Bank roof underground tunnel, platform curved away left out of sight. Rumble and roar and screech of distant trains like beasts subsiding 'Mind the gap!' loud voice deeply resonating, giggles and mimicry from tourists. Reflections of fluorescent strip bisecting the ceiling, wall tiles below white painted plaster with mouldy patches breaking through. The rails singing before train erupts from the dark mouth of the tunnel towards us. DH Lawrence would have a field day. I'm going to treat this audition as practice and fun.

****

Gabriel

Gin's been fighting – always expensive.
'The losers get bitten in the tail, he's a winner. You're brave
aren't you?' observed the vet admiringly, while Gin purred
courageously at him with a noise reminiscent of bubbling
porridge.
'There, I've drained the abcess [again], you'll need to do it first
thing every morning.' The vet had shaved Gin's head [again].
Multifarious white scar lines criss-crossed the top of his
narrow skull.

I got the part of the vet in the TV series, so this was quite a
useful visit for research purposes. I remember Undine saying
that night in Chiswick Mall, seems a long time ago now, that
she was sure I'd be successful. I wish she was here to share
the news and celebrate with. Because she's not, although I'm
relieved to have acting work, it feels empty.

I set time aside to listen to a programme on Radio 4 last night
about brain surgery for people suffering from severe
depression or OCD. I want to find out as much as I can so
that I can help Undine if we get together again. It was very
disturbing in places, particularly the butchery used performing
clumsy frontal labotomies during the 1950s, sometimes
without anaesthetic. I became aware of the huge largely
concealed section of the population who enter hospitals, are
sectioned, and suffer in silence and isolation. People much
more capable than me, for instance, in responsible posts with
stressful careers, who become ill.

Apparently now, mental health experts can measure areas of
excessive activity in the brain. One of the experts on the
programme said that a battery-operated, specifically targeted
electrode implanted in the brain, to interrupt circuits of
unhealthy thinking and brain tissue, is the way forward. But
you have to have a small operation to replace the batteries
every six months. Is it open to abuse having a foreign body
such as that in your head? What happens if batteries aren't
available? Anyway, it apparently only helps the moods of
about a third of those suffering from depression. The rituals

of the unfortunate people with severe OCD aren't helped as dramatically and it doesn't totally remove the compulsion.

Undine likes, liked, me to kiss the middle of the top of her head. Perhaps I broke the painful circuit of thought. If I could just be with her again, I'd just keep kissing away her cares and never leave her. Now I've got work, I'd be able to pay for any treatment, if she wanted it. I'd help her all the time. I should be on top of the world now that I'm acting again, but I've only made it emotionally to the Equator. We start filming in three weeks, I won't have time to search for Undine after that.

....

I've discovered sex,' Abigail said loudly as the pasta arrived. The plates jerked in the waiter's hands beside my ear. A sea of high-lighted heads in the Chelsea restaurant swung in our direction, like wheat swaying in the wind. 'Right,' I said quietly, picking up a fork. 'Yes, I'm really good at it.' There was a loud report from cricked necks. Not only does Abigail have to be formidably focused, very successful in her academic career, but good at this as well. It brought back memories of the university Common Room. Abigail asking: 'What did you get, Bella?' 'B+' said Bella very proudly, with a big smile at us all. 'Oh, poor you,' cried Abigail, 'I got A++' She'll probably get another BA (Bedroom Antics) Hons. Better not to venture far along the acronym trail. I know she's pretty, and interested, but I want Undine.

I understand what it must feel like to be a lepidopterist, trying to catch sight of Undine, let alone pin her down. Perhaps I'll find her again on this black-puddled Winter day. Think positive, Gabriel. I'll cycle up to the heath, I know she likes going there. It won't take long and I've a couple of hours before it gets dark.

****

Undine

I miss Gabriel so much. I hadn't realised how many things would remind me of him, I can't listen to opera music without crying. Matilda brought round a lovely card showing a photo of a sun-rise he'd taken. I know she thinks I should give him another chance, but it's all too much to cope with. Better I get over him now than later, when it might be even worse.

I keep doing things as though Gabriel's watching. It feels pointless dressing-up or taking a pride in my appearance, but I do it anyway, hoping I'll run into him. I imagine that happening a lot, although I try not to, and of him telling me it was all lies about the party and that he still loves me. Thank goodness I'm still able to concentrate at work. The routine, plus being distracted by the others in the office from my thoughts helps a lot. It's bliss enjoying work for once, and I still get pleasure from the knowledge that I'm skilled at the job.

I think that work improving my self-confidence is helping me to cope with learning more about OCD. There was a programme on the radio the other evening about a current theory of carrying out brain surgery to treat severe, intractable OCD. They mention, for example, anterior capsulotomy, and cingulotomy, I remember something about this from the books I read.***
Following such 'intervention' – don't you just love the bland language – I think they recommend a programme of behavioural therapy and drugs. They say that the operation isn't curative, but puts the patient in a position that is more amenable to such techniques. Must be awful if after all that, you prove to be one of the percentage of OCD sufferers for whom treatment of any kind just doesn't help.

I read somewhere that the hallmark of an obsessive phobia is not a direct fear of a given object or situation, but rather of imagined circumstances arising from them. That explains why I can deal with a flood fairly efficiently but am unable to tear myself away from staring at taps. Actually I'm practicing just looking once, then walking away. It's tough, but I'm getting much better at it and feeling better afterwards. Whatever happens, I'm going to try not to take drugs for my OCD. In fact, I'm also trying now to eat sensibly, although it still goes by the wayside if I'm very miserable. I hold it together at work as I've said, but week-ends are very long at the moment, although I'm managing to stay away from alcohol. I can't believe Gabriel did that, but why would Torquil lie?

Good news: I have discovered that the risk of an OCD sufferer actually performing the feared act of murder, rape, paedophilia etcetera, is rare. Fortunate that, or prisons would become so crowded that inmate and public would eventually be forced to reverse accommodation. The prisoners could move out into community housing to have, in Woolf's immortal phrase, a room of one's own, and the general public would whizz thankfully into prison for some space. It would precipitate even more Interior Design television programmes: Cell Block Marbling perhaps, or Illusions of Space using *Teint de Ivoire*, would grip the contained population nightly. Meanwhile criminals would be suffering from agoraphobia…

****

Gabriel

I had a dream that I was hunting – bizarre.   I was like one of those guys in the African bush around the time of the Boer War. My heart was beating loudly and I was trying to hold my breath to quieten it down. I was staring down from my hide in a tree at a timid and wary creature that I was trying to shoot, far below me. It looked around, I was terrified that it would look up but it returned to grazing, halting often to lift it's head and stare about. Then it walked over to the tree and began looking intently at the bark. I suddenly had the feeling that it knew I was there, but it just sniffed delicately down the trunk to the grass and flowers growing around the base. It lay down and I still couldn't force myself to shoot it. After a quarter of an hour I had to move, cramp was clutching at muscles in my calf. As blossom drifted down from the branches, the unicorn looked up, straight into my eyes, then rose unhurriedly and wandered away. Lower branches, then grass brushed against my hunting boots as I descended and

followed. I dropped the gun to the ground. Then it was as if I
was nostalgically watching the closing credits of an old techni-
coloured Hollywood film: the camera panned back and the
two beings gradually diminished in size, walking peaceably
towards distant blue hills lying beneath an over-arching
rainbow.

....

I've found her! It's Sunday. A guy was coming out of the
front door as I approached, so I entered the squat and looked
round until I found her door ajar. Undine was sitting on the
floor of her room surrounded by open tins of food. A half-
eaten loaf of new bread was on a plate next to her.
'Oh hello,' she said, white-faced, not noticeably put out at
being caught in the midst of an eating binge. Nevertheless
she looked thin, clad in a dressing-gown and with her hair
scraped back into a band.
'How did you find me?'
'I persuaded Chloris and Matilda finally to tell me, didn't you
get my messages?'
'Don't you just adore eating?' she asked coldly, peeling a
banana. 'It's the best thing in the world. One wishes that one
could just taste all the food in the world, to see which is
nicest, without actually having to swallow it and put on
weight.'
'You could spit it out,'
'No I couldn't.' Her hand began shaking and she blindly put
the banana back on the plate. Tears poured down her face, I
felt dreadful. I daringly took her in my arms, she didn't
respond for a minute, then hugged me back. Undine's face
was wet against my neck.
'I promise nothing happened at that party,' I said breathlessly,
I thought my heart would break. 'I didn't find out what Torquil
told you until afterwards,' I leaned back to look into her eyes,
'You do believe me don't you, little one?'
'I want to, he was so pleased to tell me. He must really hate
me, and I'd thought Torquil quite liked me really.' She
sobbed, wiping her eyes on her sleeve.
'He's not important now, Torquil's a total jealous fuck-head-'
'You just swore, so did the man on the 'phone! I thought it
wasn't you because you don't swear, oh Gabriel-'

'Undine, Undine! It wasn't me on the 'phone.'
'Do you promise?' She stopped crying and looked panic-stricken instead.
'I promise,' I said firmly, gently rubbing her cold hands. 'And I do swear occasionally when someone's been an idiot like Torquil. He's not important, he doesn't live on the boat any more.'
I looked at her hopefully, but she was looking down. She freed her hands and began pulling at a loose thread on her dressing-gown.
'Oh please, please come back Undine, you don't know how lonely it's been without you. Even Tonic has given up eating.'
I knelt back on my heels and found I'd put my knee in a cake. We laughed shakily. I sank down onto the double bed and began to brush it off. 'Do you want one? I don't want any more.' She held out the packet of sponge cakes.
'No thanks.'
The gloomy room was suddenly lit by a violet flash, a minute later thunder rumbled in the distance as we listened. A few drops of rain spattered in a grey flurry against the sash windows.
'Really, did nothing happen at the party?' She stared at me.
'Nothing happened. Cross my heart and hope to die.'
'Why did Torquil lie?'
'I think he thought he was in love with me, he's living properly with Chris now.'
'Oh, I'm glad Chris is all right.'
'They're good,' I said suddenly, noticing new drawings stuck to the wall. I stood up. It's a new architectural plan of Einstein Road, the whole house, done in axonometric. I peer down into the rooms from above. There's Undine's room, the sitting room, the hall, all radiating a glow of bright colour. She's even accurately depicted Matilda and Chloris in there, Chloris cooking. Nearby on the wall, on another sheet of A3, is a plan of *The Ark*, I look anxiously among the perfect ink lines to see who inhabits the vessel. One cat: Camberwell, Undine's even captured his peevish expression. There's me, Tonic and Leo … And Undine, sitting reading on the sofa in the sitting-room with Gin.
'In fact it's fantastic!'
'Thanks,' says Undine, looking thrilled. She blushed: 'I do have some talent you know.'

'I know, sorry darling, I just didn't know the developments in this latest one. Now can we go back to that one you have for making me the happiest man alive?'

'Oh, okay then,' she said with mock-reluctance.

'Come here you!'

Pause

'I love you to infinity...'

'Times infinity,'

'Plus one.'

Pause

'Times a million. Oh, there is one thing you have to promise me young Undine.'

'What?' She looked momentarily apprehensive.

'Never, ever, to leave me again - in any way. You *promise* to talk to me first before you even think of it.'

'I promise, angel.' She hugged me.

'What? To leave me, or not?'

She giggled: 'Not to. I wanted to talk to you Gabriel ... I missed you terribly-

Pause

'I leueuve you!'

'Plus two.'

Pause

'Squared.'

Very long pause. I can't multi-task after all.

....

Undine can though. I was waiting for her with Liam at Pickwicks the following week, she was about half an hour late. I make allowances for her being late because of the OCD, but she's usually on time. We were just finishing off our pints when Undine came in, exuding vivid excitement. Liam blushed - he always does when he sees beautiful girls.

'Hi Gabriel, guess what? I've got a surprise for you outside,' she said all in one breath, before giving me a warm kiss. 'Hi Liam.' She beamed at him; he positively simpered. I followed her through the crowd, leaving Liam to guard our seats. Outside, tied to a lamppost with her woolly scarf, was my bicycle.

'Oh darling, thanks! Thank-you. Where did you find it?'

'I was on my way here, and I saw this gang of kids on bikes, virtually invisible in the dark. I thought one of the bikes looked like yours and when this boy cycled under a streetlamp I was sure. So I ran across the road, his mates saw me coming before he did, all their faces changed. He was just beginning to accelerate away and I grabbed him by the waistband of his trousers. It was really hard holding onto him and the bike, he kept struggling to get away on it. Luckily his friends didn't interfere, just stood around in a semi-circle, apart from one little beast, the ringleader I think. He was the oldest, he kept making nasty comments.' She stopped for breath, I gave her a hug.

'That's so lovely, and brave, of you doing that for me.'

'I just kept shouting, "That's my boyfriend's bike!" I think they were quite scared.'

Anyway, I wasn't strong enough to drag him and the bike to the Station so we had a bit of an impasse. Thank goodness this really nice Italian woman stopped and said: 'You give that young lady back her bike,' and this boy started swearing his head off at her. Then I got angry all over again and gave him a bit of a shake, and said: "Stop swearing at her, you!"

He shouted: "I'm not 'you', I'm Joshua!" They all gasped and Joshua looked stunned. It was quite funny. There was this sudden silence, then two policemen crossed the road, walking slowly and grinning, and the boys shot off in all directions. Joshua raced off down that side street.'

I kissed her gratefully, 'I think you've done absolutely brilliantly, darling.'

'I do too,' Undine said, beaming joyously, 'but they've really wrecked it.' Her face suddenly clouded with anxiety and she drew back from me: 'Do you think Joshua is all right? Perhaps I hurt him.'

'No, you didn't, or he wouldn't have run off so fast. Anyway, even if you did, which you didn't, I'll stand by you.'

'Thanks,' her face cleared.

'Much more importantly, how did they manage to do this much damage in three weeks?'

I inspected the bike closely, it looked as though it'd had a close encounter with a lorry. Never mind, I can repair it.

****

Romance

In the evenings, Ursula was fussed over during the apres-ski gatherings now taking place in the Bar. While everyone around her enthusiastically drank and related their progress on the ski slopes, she listened and resisted offers of beer, and other more flirtatious offers. Ursula blossomed. She felt as though she was now enjoying a youthful time she hadn't been able to before. She avoided alcohol: both her parents had drunk rather too much at different times and she liked to be in command of herself. Perhaps she had exercised too much control and caution, Ursula sometimes thought. Never mind, her life was opening up enough now.

Towards the end of the holiday, Ursula began to consider putting together her sketches and paintings into a portfolio. Several people had now commented favourably on her work. She remembered there were a lot of canvases tucked away in a large cupboard - some she hadn't looked at for several years. Maybe she could even exhibit them somewhere? It would be wonderful to earn money from something she enjoyed doing so much. Sorry as she would be to leave the Alps, she looked forward to returning to London.

****

Undine

I'm walking out of the usual Tube station, it seems very brightly-lit, like a strange stage set. I deftly avoid the loitering people waiting with joyous anticipation for friends. Others are talking to themselves but, one supposes, really to mobile 'phones. Anyone can resemble a nutter; in fact at least one in four of us is one at some point in our lives apparently. The clever and strong trick is to be one and not hide it. I can see strangers crying out for joy, hugging and kissing each other. Eventually they walk away towards the brightly-lit shops and cafes, bars and restaurants. I know, because I stand watching.

Now I'm moving right, along the high-sided elegant street again. I take a moment to look up, the houses sail like tall ships against the scudding clouds. Quietly I walk on, dreamily I descend the narrow steps, I touch the railings even though I'm not wearing gloves.

****

Alexander

Alexander was wondering where his silver paper knife was, he'd looked for it to bring it back to the basement – first his pen and now this! It was unusual for other psychotherapists who worked from the consulting room to borrow one another's things. Sitting on the arm of the chair, he reached for a pencil to make a note on his pad. As he read, he heard a noise outside on the steps. He wasn't expecting any patients today: it had better not be that pestiferous gang of boys on bikes again. Alexander added a couple of reminders to his shopping list. The lead broke and he threw the pencil down irritably. Looking up, he saw a distorted figure through the frosted glass window, gliding down the steps outside. Surprised, he rose and walked cautiously across the quiet room to open the door.

****

Undine

Alexander's just your normal fucked-up human being, as he said during that first session, aeons ago. Poor thing, he looked quite scared when I breezed in and kissed him good-bye this afternoon. His body felt rigid when I hugged him, I didn't realise he's so muscular. I don't find him sexy any more, a bit too flashy somehow. He's back to normal, apart from looking slightly nervous. Whatever briefly upset him and his appearance has obviously been vanquished. I bravely returned his pen and apologised, now I've finished with it. I've written the 'Taurus' chapter.

The basement looked as though a bomb had hit it, speedy removal was obviously in progress. The curtains were open and the room looked forlorn in the clear wintry light. Files were scattered around on the desk, chairs and floor. There were pale squares on the wallpaper where pictures had been removed; these were now stacked against the wall. A couple of boxes were open containing objects wrapped in newspaper. The surfaces of the desk and bureau were dusty and empty, with shiny areas where books and things had stood – seemingly for eternity in that cosy lamplight. Alexander's computer was on the floor, wires trailing. A couple of piles of books stood like tower blocks on the floor, tied up with string. The carpet, I could now see, was stained in places and fraying at the edges. The sofa sagged in the centre. The armchair in which I'd first sat - it seems so long ago, but was only last March - was worn thin and shiny along the arms and headrest. Absorbing these new impressions, I forgot to tell Alexander about Marius acting strangely. I don't think it matters. Vivienne reported at the February meeting last week (when to her surprise, I paid my rent – and I've repaid Chloris) that Marius's room is available. Apparently he's gone to Australia for an indefinite period. Good riddance.

****

Gabriel

'I know.' I smiled across at Undine, she was lying reading on the sofa, with Gin beside her.
'What do you mean, you know? We searched for her for ages!' Torquil sounded put out.
'Undine looked at me enquiringly, Gin pushed his nose against her book.
'Torquil. He and Chris have been hunting for you,' I said, hand over the receiver. Her eyebrows shot up.
I removed my hand: 'I know because I found Undine myself last week, and she's here on the boat with me right now.'
'I'm glad, I'm *really* sorry about what I did.'

'Right, Torquil.'
'I am! I don't know what I was thinking of.'
'I do, you were being a complete and utter selfish shit!'
Undine and Gin looked across at me apprehensively, I
realised I was shouting.
'It won't happen again-'
'No, it won't. Why are you ringing anyway?'
'Well I felt bad, being so happy with Chris, I love him you
know.' I snorted.
'All right Gabriel, as much as I can love anybody!'
'That's better. Before you go on, you can apologise to
Undine.'
'Yes, yes, of course I will.' Love *has* changed him.
'Do you want to talk to Torquil? He wants to say he's sorry,
darling. You don't have to.'
I looked at Undine, she reached out reluctantly for the 'phone.
'Yes?' she said, holding it gingerly.
I could Torquil's squeaks coming from the mouthpiece for a
while.
'All right, yes' said Undine eventually. Then, 'I'll ask Gabriel.
[to me] Do you mind if he and Chris come round?'
'Do you?'
'I suppose not, I'd like to see Chris anyway.'

....

It was lovely to see Chris, and tolerable seeing Torquil for the
first time since all the upset. Chris does seem to be good for
him, Torquil is calmer and happier. Apparently Chris wants to
sponsor my idea for individual cat flaps, with twee curtains,
and an option of cat-brushing, paw-cleaning entrance. Good
news does happen in threes, because Undine's pregnant - it
must have happened in the land-based shed that day in the
rain. But we're not telling anybody until she's had all the tests
– that's her decision, I just want to shout it to the world from
the deck.
I thought she might throw up when Chris was discussing
whether he should have laser eye-treatment and Torquil said:
'I've *told* him, you lose your night vision, and they cut a flap in
your eyeball they don't close up, like a cat flap... Have I said
something?'

****

Gabriel

We burnt Undine's old diaries in April on the allotment, soon after Undine moved in. The cats thought it was great, sitting in a semi-circle around the conflagration. Finn arranged boat insurance through a mate for us, but we visit Matilda and Chloris a lot, in lieu of living round the corner from them at Camden Lock. Undine insists on visiting the cockatiels at the same time, chatting away to them at their new home in a huge aviary at Regents Park, in this case not killing two birds with one stone.

I had a day off from filming last week and I planted vegetables and Undine flowers, in a new bed we dug together a while back on the allotment. Florence and Maisie are coming to dinner again when the vegetables are ready for harvesting. Undine was having difficulty reaching round her bump to put the seedlings in the earth, which made us laugh. It's great that the land already has an apple tree, bees and clusters of roses slowly unfurling over the shed door. I even spotted a grass snake sliding peaceably along one of the mossy paths.

THE END

Bibliography

*Zak et al., 1988; De Veaugh-Geiss, Katz and Landau, 1989; Greist,1990a

**The Treatment of Anxiety Disorders - G Andrews, M Creamer, R Crino

***C Hunt, L Lampe and A Page. Second Ed. Cambridge Univ. Press, 2003

Treatment Plans and Interventions for Depression & Anxiety Disorders – R L Leahy & S J Holland, 2000

Cognitive Therapy:100 Key Points and Techniques – M Neenan & W Dryden

Fears and Phobias - Isaac M Marks, 1969

Linda Goodman's Sun Signs – Bantam Books, 1968.